ACID REFLUX COOKBOOK

Low Acid Recipes to Put Gerd or Acid Reflux Under Control

(Treatment and Cure of Gerd and Gastritis on a Acid Reflux Diet)

Elisabeth Schrom

Published by Alex Howard

© **Elisabeth Schrom**

All Rights Reserved

Acid Reflux Cookbook: Low Acid Recipes to Put Gerd or Acid Reflux Under Control (Treatment and Cure of Gerd and Gastritis on a Acid Reflux Diet)

ISBN 978-1-77485-001-5

Legal & Disclaimer

The information contained in this book is not designed to replace or take the place of any form of medicine or professional medical advice. The information in this book has been provided for educational and entertainment purposes only.

Table of contents

Part 1

Introduction

Acid reflux is a painful condition caused by stomach acid going up the esophagus. The intensity of acid reflux can vary from person to person, and it is important to always ask your doctor about the best treatment options for you. With that little disclaimer out of the way, there are ways you can get relief from your acid reflux symptoms naturally, through changes in your diet.

The type of foods you eat in your diet is a very important factor for controlling acid reflux, some foods will make your acid reflux worse while others will help you get relief from your acid reflux symptoms. Below are some quick tips for helping you control your acid reflux.

Foods That Can Make Your Acid Reflux Worse:

- Foods that are high in fat or deep fried

- Fruits that contain high amounts of acid, like lemons, oranges and tomatoes

- Spicy foods

- Foods high in sugar (desserts, and chocolate)

- High amounts of dairy

- Onions and garlic

Foods That Can Help Relieve Acid Reflux:

- Oats and whole grains

- Low acid fruits like bananas and apples

- Avocados

- Ginger

- Green vegetables and cauliflower

- Potatoes (not fried)

- Low fat meats

It is important to remember that some foods on this list may be okay for some people, but will trigger acid reflux for others. This is why it is important to talk to your doctor about your condition, so they can determine what foods you should and shouldn't be eating.

Chapter 1: GERD Diet Breakfast Recipes

Banana Oatmeal Pancakes

Ingredients

1/2 cup oatmeal, uncooked

3 egg whites

1 medium banana, lightly mashed

vanilla (to taste)

Directions

Mix together oatmeal, egg whites and banana, add vanilla to taste (optional).

Spray large skillet with cooking spray. Cook until browned on each side.

Makes 4 pancakes.

Applesauce Oat Breakfast Muffins

Ingredients

1 cup rolled oats

1 cup 1% milk

1 cup whole wheat flour

1 teaspoon baking powder

1/2 teaspoon baking soda

1/2 cup brown sugar

1/2 cup applesauce

1 egg

Directions

Place oats in a small bowl, pour in buttermilk. Let sit for two hours at room temperature.

Preheat oven to 375 degrees F (190 degrees C). Grease 12 muffin cups or line with paper muffin liners.

In a large bowl, stir together whole wheat flour, baking powder, baking soda and brown sugar. Stir in oat/buttermilk mixture, applesauce and egg; mix well. Pour batter into prepared muffin cups.

Bake in preheated oven for 30 minutes, until a toothpick inserted into center of muffin comes out clean.

Banana Oatmeal Muffins

Ingredients

1 cup quick oats

1 cup whole wheat flour

1/2 tsp salt

1 tsp baking powder

1 tsp baking soda

1/2 cup brown sugar

2 egg whites

1/2 cup natural apple sauce

1/2 cup 1% milk

1/2 cup nonfat yogurt

7 tbsp whole ground flaxseed meal

2 ripe bananas

Directions

In a bowl, soak oats in milk and yogurt with the brown sugar for about one hour.

Mash two ripe bananas, combine with applesauce and egg whites.

In a separate bowl combine flour, salt, baking powder, baking soda, salt and ground flax seed.

Add banana mixture to the soaked oats, mix well, add in dry mixture.

Careful not to over mix muffin batter or muffins will be too tough.

Preheat the oven to 400F. Spray muffin pans lightly with cooking spray.

Bake for approximately 25 minutes or until done.

Coconut Oatmeal

Ingredients

3 1/2 cups vanilla soy milk

1/4 teaspoon salt

2 cups rolled oats

1/4 cup pure maple syrup

1/3 cup dried cranberries

1/3 cup sweetened flaked coconut

1 (8 ounce) container plain yogurt (optional)

3 tablespoons honey (optional)

Directions

Pour the milk and salt into a saucepan, and bring to a boil. Stir in the oats, maple syrup, , and cranberries. Return to a boil, then reduce heat to medium.

Cook for 5 minutes. Stir in coconut, and let stand until it reaches your desired thickness.

Spoon into serving bowls, and top with yogurt and honey, if desired.

Banana Oatmeal Breakfast Smoothie

Ingredients

1 banana, broken into chunks

1/2 cup plain low-fat yogurt

1/2 cup almond milk

1/4 cup old-fashioned rolled oats

2 teaspoons honey

Directions

Combine banana, yogurt, almond milk, oats, and honey, in a blender; blend until smooth.

Zucchini Muffins

Ingredients

2 cups whole wheat flour

1 tablespoon baking powder

1/2 teaspoon salt

3/4 cup nonfat milk

2 egg whites

1/4 cup vegetable oil

1/4 cup honey

1 cup grated zucchini

Directions

Preheat oven to 375 degrees F (190 degrees C). Grease muffin tins lightly with oil or spray with a non-stick cooking spray.

Combine whole wheat flour, baking powder, salt and ground cinnamon, mix thoroughly.

Mix the milk, slightly beaten egg whites, oil, honey and shredded zucchini together. Pour into the dry

ingredients and stir until just barely moistened. Batter should be lumpy. Fill muffin tins 2/3 full with batter.

Bake at 375 degrees F (190 degrees C) for 20 minutes or until lightly browned.

Coconut Granola Breakfast

Ingredients

8 cups quick-cooking oats

1 cup oat bran

1 cup unsweetened flaked coconut

1/2 cup coconut milk

1/4 cup virgin coconut oil

1/4 cup vegetable oil

1/2 cup barley malt syrup or maltose syrup

1/2 cup honey

1 teaspoon vanilla extract

1/2 cup dried cranberries

Directions

Preheat the oven to 350 degrees F (175 degrees C). In a large bowl, stir together the oats, oat bran, and coconut. Divide between two large baking sheets, and spread into an even layer.

Bake for 7 or 8 minutes in the preheated oven, until lightly toasted. Allow to cool for a few minutes, then return to the large bowl.

While the oats are toasting, combine the coconut milk, coconut oil, vegetable oil, malt syrup and honey in a saucepan. Cook over medium heat, stirring until it comes to a boil. Boil for 2 minutes. Remove from heat, and stir in the vanilla.

Pour the syrup over the granola in the bowl, and stir until the dry **ingredients** are fully coated. Divide between the two baking sheets, and spread evenly.

Bake for 8 minutes in the preheated oven, or until fragrant and toasted. Cool in the pans, then mix in the dried cranberries. Store in an airtight container at room temperature.

Oatmeal Mango Porridge

Ingredients

1/2 cup quick oats

1/4 cup low-fat milk

1/3 cup low-fat plain yogurt

1/8 teaspoon almond extract

1/2 cup diced mango

1 teaspoon honey

1 teaspoon chia seeds

Directions

Add oats to your container of choice and pour in milk and low-fat yogurt.

Mix in almond extract. Add a layer of mango. Top off with a drizzle of honey and chia seeds.

Place in fridge overnight, and serve the following day.

Applesauce Pancakes

Ingredients

1 1/4 cups unbleached all-purpose flour

1/2 cup whole wheat flour

1/4 cup wheat germ

2 teaspoons baking powder

1 tablespoon canola oil

3 egg yolks

5 egg whites

1/2 cup unsweetened applesauce

1/2 cup skim milk, or as needed

1 teaspoon vegetable oil

Directions

In a large bowl, stir together the all-purpose flour, whole wheat flour, wheat germ, and baking powder. Make a well in the center, and stir in the egg yolks, applesauce and milk until fairly smooth. If the batter seems too thick, stir in more milk.

In a separate bowl, whip the egg whites with an electric mixer to soft peaks. Fold egg whites into the batter, just until blended.

Heat the oil in a large skillet over medium heat. Scoop large spoonfuls of batter onto the hot pan, and fry until bubbles appear on the surface.

Flip and cook until browned on the other side. Continue with remaining batter.

Sweet Potato Porridge

Ingredients

1/3 cup water

1/4 cup plain fat-free Greek yogurt

1/4 cup old-fashioned rolled oats

1/2 scoop vanilla protein powder

1 tablespoon ground flax seed

1 1/2 teaspoons chia seeds

1/4 cup sweet potato puree

2 tablespoons water

Directions

Stir 1/3 cup water, yogurt, oats, protein powder, ground flax seed, and chia seeds, together in a bowl; add sweet potatoes and 2 tablespoons water and stir until well mixed.

Refrigerate 8 hours to overnight.

Oatmeal Yogurt Pancakes

Ingredients

1/2 cup oats

1/2 cup fat-free Greek yogurt

4 egg whites

1/2 tsp baking powder

1/2 tsp vanilla

1 tbsp sugar

1/2 tsp cinnamon

Directions

Blend everything except the oats. Once you have a smooth liquid, add the oats and blend until just mixed.

Let the batter rest for 5 minutes.

Coat a skillet with nonstick spray, then place over medium-high heat.

Add 1/4 cup batter to the pan at a time, flipping when the pancake starts to bubble. Remove from heat once fully cooked.

Oatmeal Yogurt Muffins

Ingredients

2 cups flour

1 cup quick oats

1/2 cup brown sugar

4 tsp baking powder

2 tsp baking soda

1 tsp salt

1 1/3 cup fat free plain yogurt

1 1/3 cup water

Directions

Mix flour, oats, sugar, baking powder, baking soda and salt. Mix yogurt with water.

Add wet **ingredients** to flour mixture, stirring until just blended.

Bake at 400F, 18-20 minutes.

Chapter 2: GERD Diet Lunch

Creamy Carrot Ginger Soup

Ingredients

4 cups baby carrots

4 cups low sodium chicken stock

2 cups water

1 (14 ounce) can coconut milk

1 (1 inch) piece fresh ginger, peeled and minced

1 teaspoon sea salt, or more to taste

1 teaspoon dried cilantro

Directions

Place baby carrots in a large pot with enough water to cover by several inches; bring to a boil and cook until tender, about 10 minutes; drain and return carrots to the pot.

Pour chicken stock, 2 cups water, and coconut milk over the carrots; add, ginger, and sea salt.

Bring the mixture to a boil, reduce heat to low, and cook at a simmer for 45 minutes.

Pour soup into a blender no more than half full. Cover and hold lid down; pulse a few times before leaving on to blend.

Puree in batches until smooth and return to the pot. Stir cilantro through the soup; season with salt.

Creamy White Bean Pumpkin Soup

Ingredients

1 sprays olive oil cooking spray, or enough to coat pot

15 oz canned pumpkin

3 1/2 cup fat-free chicken broth

15 1/2 oz canned white beans, rinsed and drained

1/4 tsp ground oregano

1/8 tsp table salt, or to taste

Directions

Spray crockpot with cooking spray (1-2 seconds).

Combine all **ingredients** in crockpot. Cover and cook on low setting for 8-10 hours.

Savory Butternut Squash Soup

Ingredients

1 tablespoon butter

1 tablespoon olive oil

4 cups low sodium chicken broth

1 butternut squash - peeled, seeded, and cubed

1 (1 inch) piece fresh ginger, peeled and grated

1 teaspoon ground cumin (optional)

salt to taste

2 cups water

1 cup quinoa

1 tablespoon butter

Directions

Heat 1 tablespoon butter and olive oil together in a skillet over medium heat; Add chicken broth, butternut squash, ginger, and cumin. Simmer over medium heat until squash is very soft, about 20 minutes.

Pour squash mixture into a blender no more than half full. Cover and hold lid down; pulse a few times before leaving on to blend.

Puree in batches until smooth.

Bring salted water and quinoa to a boil in a saucepan. Reduce heat to medium-low, cover, and simmer until quinoa is tender and water has been absorbed, 15 to 20 minutes.

Stir 1 tablespoon butter into cooked quinoa and season with salt. Spoon quinoa into soup.

Brown Rice And Lentil Soup

Ingredients

9 cups water

3 tablespoons vegetable bouillon powder

1 1/2 cups lentils

1 cup brown rice

3 carrots chopped into medium-small pieces

2 celery stalks, chopped

1 tsp dry coriander

1 tsp dry basil

1 tsp thyme

1 bay leaf

Directions

Add all **ingredients** into a pot and cook, covered, for one hour. Add salt to taste.

Thai Coconut Chicken Ginger Soup

Ingredients

3 cups coconut milk

2 cups water

1/2 pound skinless, boneless chicken breast halves - cut into thin strips

3 tablespoons minced fresh ginger root

1 tablespoon chopped fresh cilantro

Directions

Pour the coconut milk and water into a saucepan, and bring to a boil. Add the chicken strips, and reduce heat to medium.

Simmer for about 3 minutes, just until the chicken is cooked through. Stir in the ginger, sprinkle in cilantro and serve.

Avocado Corn Salad

Ingredients

1 cup cut corn, fresh or frozen

1 tablespoon vegetable oil

2 tablespoons water

1 teaspoon ground cumin (optional)

1 avocado

salt

chopped fresh cilantro

Directions

In a large skillet, add corn, oil, water, cumin.

Over medium heat, cook, covered, for 5 minutes or until the corn is tender.

Uncover and continue to cook for a few minutes to evaporate the excess moisture.

Set skillet aside to cool. Slice the avocado in half lengthwise and remove the pit.

Peel the avocado and chop into 1/2 inch pieces and place in a large bowl.

Add the cooked corn; stir to combine. Sprinkle fresh chopped cilantro on top.

Sweet Potato Ginger Bisque

Ingredients

1 (2 pound) butternut squash - peeled, seeded, and cut into large chunks

4 sweet potatoes, peeled and cut into chunks

1 (2 inch) piece fresh ginger, peeled and finely chopped

1 1/2 quarts water, or amount to cover

1 cup plain low fat yogurt

salt to taste

Directions

Place the squash, sweet potatoes, and ginger in a large pot. Pour in enough water to cover the vegetables.

Bring to simmer over medium heat, and cook until vegetables are tender and can be easily pierced with a fork, 30 to 45 minutes.

Remove pot from heat. Place soup in batches into a blender or the bowl of a food process. Pulse until smooth.

Return soup to pot, and whisk in yogurt. Season with salt to taste. If necessary, reheat soup over low heat, but do not allow to boil.

Wild Rice Vegetable Soup

Ingredients

3/4 cup lentils, sorted and rinsed

3/4 cup diced carrot

3/4 cup diced celery

1/4 cup wild rice

1 teaspoon dried oregano

1/4 teaspoon dried thyme

5 cups water

4 teaspoons vegetable bouillon seasoning

1 bay leaf

1 tablespoon apple cider vinegar

1/4 cup minced fresh parsley

2 tablespoons minced fresh basil (optional)

Directions

Combine all **ingredients** on the list through till bayleaf in a large pot. Bring to a boil, then simmer until lentils and rice are tender, 35-45 minutes.

Remove the bay leaf. Scoop out about two cups of the soup and blend well in the blender. Return the blended soup to the pot.

Stir in the apple cider vinegar, the fresh parsley and basil if using. Serve hot.

Tuna Spinach Salad

Ingredients

1 (5 ounce) can tuna in water, drained

1/3 cup dried cranberries

1/2 apple, cut into 1/4-inch pieces

2 tablespoons light mayonnaise

sea salt to taste

4 cups chopped fresh spinach

Directions

Mix tuna, cranberries, apple, mayonnaise, sea salt, together in a bowl; refrigerate 1 hour.

Put 2 cups spinach on each of 2 plates. Top spinach with about half the tuna salad.

Chapter 3: GERD Diet Dinner Recipes

Grilled Ginger Salmon

Ingredients

1/4 cup light soy sauce

1 1/2 tablespoons honey

1 tablespoon grated fresh ginger

1 pound salmon fillets

1 teaspoon sesame oil

2 teaspoons sesame seeds

Directions

Whisk soy sauce, honey, and ginger together in a bowl until marinade is evenly mixed. Set aside 1/4 of the marinade.

Place salmon fillets in shallow dish; pour the remaining marinade over the salmon. Cover dish with plastic wrap and refrigerate for 5 minutes.

Heat sesame oil in a large skillet over medium-high heat.

Remove salmon from marinade, shaking to remove excess marinade, and place, skin-side up, into the hot oil; cook for 4 minutes. Discard unused marinade in the shallow dish.

Flip salmon and drizzle the reserved 1/4 of the marinade over salmon; sprinkle with sesame seeds.

Cook until fish flakes easily with a fork, 5 to 7 minutes. Flip salmon, remove skin, and cook 1 minute more.

Broccoli And Ginger Chicken Stir Fry

Ingredients

2 tablespoons olive oil

2 large boneless, skinless chicken breasts, cubed

1/4 cup honey

2 tablespoons finely chopped ginger

1 large head broccoli, cut into florets

1/2 cup honey

Directions

Heat olive oil in a skillet or wok over medium heat. Add chicken cubes, 1/4 cup honey, and ginger.

Cook and stir until chicken is golden brown, about 10 minutes. Add broccoli, and remaining 1/2 cup honey.

Cover and cook over medium-high heat until broccoli is tender, 5 to 10 minutes, stirring occasionally.

Grilled Sesame Chicken

Ingredients

6 skinless chicken thighs

1 tablespoon minced fresh ginger root

1 tablespoon black bean sauce

1 teaspoon sesame oil

Directions

Place thighs in a bowl, add ginger, black bean sauce, and sesame oil. Stir well until completely coated. Marinate in the refrigerator for 2 hours.

Grill over medium heat until no longer pink but still juicy, about 20 minutes, turning only once.

Chicken Barley Soup

Ingredients

8 cups water

2 pounds chicken thighs, or more to taste

1 1/2 cups chopped carrots

1 cup chopped celery

3/4 cup pearl barley

3 bay leaves

1 cube chicken bouillon, or more to taste

1 teaspoon poultry seasoning

1 teaspoon rubbed sage

1 teaspoon salt, or to taste

Directions

Combine water, chicken thighs, and bay leaves in a large stock pot; bring to a boil, reduce heat to low, place a cover on the pot, and cook at a simmer until the chicken is tender, about 30 minutes.

Remove chicken to a cutting board to cool. Remove and discard bones, skin, and fat from chicken. Cut remaining meat into bite-sized pieces.

Cool broth until the fat congeals on the surface. Skim and discard fat.

Return soup to heat; add carrots, celery, pearl barley, bay leaves, chicken bouillon, poultry seasoning, sage, salt.

Bring the soup to a boil, reduce heat to low, place cover on the pot, and simmer until the barley is cooked and the vegetables are tender, 60 to 90 minutes.

Bok Choy Soup

Ingredients

1 tablespoon vegetable oil

6 cups water

4 teaspoons chicken broth

6 small potatoes, diced

4 carrots, sliced

6 large bok choy ribs with leaves, finely chopped

2 stalks celery, sliced

2 skinless, boneless chicken breast halves, cut into 1/2-inch cubes and cooked

Directions

Heat vegetable oil in a large stockpot over medium heat. Add water, chicken broth, potatoes, carrots, bok choy, and celery; bring to a boil. Reduce heat and simmer until vegetables are slightly tender, about 10 minutes.

Add cooked chicken; continue simmering for 10 more minutes.

Chicken Vegetable Soup

Ingredients

1 whole chicken, quartered

water, to cover

1 stalk celery with leaves, cut into chunks

3 cubes chicken bouillon

1/4 cup chopped fresh basil

1/4 cup chopped fresh parsley

2 Yukon Gold potatoes, diced

2 kohlrabi bulbs, peeled and diced

2 carrots, sliced

1 large turnip, diced

1/2 medium head cabbage, chopped

2 ears sweet corn, cut from cob

4 ounces fresh green beans, trimmed

Directions

Put chicken pieces in a large stockpot; pour enough water over chicken to cover completely. Add celery, bouillon cubes, basil, parsley, salt, to the pot; bring to a simmer over medium-high heat.

Cook at a simmer until the chicken is cooked through and tender, about 1 hour.

Remove and discard celery chunks. Remove chicken to a cutting board to cool; cut as much meat as possible from the bones and chop roughly. Return chicken to stock.

Stir potatoes, kohlrabi, carrots, and turnip into the soup; cook until the vegetables are tender, about 20 minutes.

Add cabbage, corn, green beans; cook until the green beans are tender, 7 to 10 minutes more.

Chicken And Mushroom Barley Soup

Ingredients

2 tablespoons olive oil

1 cup chopped celery

4 cups sliced fresh mushrooms

1 cup chopped carrots

5 cups diced red potatoes

3 cups chopped cooked chicken

2 1/2 quarts chicken broth

1 cup quick-cooking barley

2 tablespoons butter

1/2 cup chopped fresh parsley

Directions

Heat the oil in a large stock pot over medium heat. Cook celery, mushrooms, in olive oil until tender.

Stir in carrots, potatoes, chicken, and broth. Bring to a boil, then stir in barley. Reduce heat, cover, and simmer 20 minutes.

Remove from heat, and stir in butter, parsley. Season with salt to taste.

Sesame Honey Chicken

Ingredients

6 boneless skinless chicken breast halves, pat dry with paper towels

$\frac{1}{2}$ cup honey

$\frac{1}{2}$ cup low sodium soy sauce

1 cup water

2 tablespoons cornstarch

$\frac{1}{2}$-1 teaspoon ground ginger

1 tablespoon toasted sesame seeds

Directions

Cut chicken breast into 1 inch strips or bite size pieces. Heat a large non-stick skillet that has been sprayed with cooking spray, over medium-high heat.

Cook chicken for about 6 minutes or until no longer pink. Mix together honey, soy sauce, water, corn starch, ginger.

Whisk until no corn starch lumps appear. Pour sauce mixture into skillet with chicken.

Cook until sauce thickens slightly, add more water if sauce is too thick.

Sprinkle with sesame seeds. Cover and simmer for 10 minutes.

Mushroom Chicken

Ingredients

4 boneless skinless chicken breasts

$\frac{1}{2}$ lb white button mushrooms, sliced thinly

1 can chicken broth, divided

$\frac{1}{2}$ cup water

3 tablespoons soya sauce, divided

3 tablespoons cornstarch

4 tablespoons water (to mix with cornstarch)

salt and pepper

Directions

Mix the cornstarch with enough water to make a thin paste.

Simmer the mushrooms in 2 tbsp soya sauce in a non-stick pan at low heat until tender. Remove mushrooms and set aside.

Add 1 tbsp soya sauce and 1 tbsp chicken broth to the pan juices and add chicken, turning to coat as much of the chicken as possible in the soya sauce.

Cook at a medium low heat until the chicken is almost done.

Mix the remaining chicken broth and 1/2 cup water (or broth) in a saucepan. Bring to a boil.

Add a few tbsp of the hot liquid to the cornstarch paste, stir until smooth and then stir into the boiling gravy until thickened.

Add the mushrooms to the gravy. Stir to mix.

Pour gravy over chicken in pan and simmer until tender.

Brown Rice Chicken Salad

Ingredients

2 tablespoons chopped fresh basil leaves

2 cups cooked chicken, cooled and coarsely chopped

1 1/2 cups cooked brown rice, cooled

1 cup fresh mango, peeled and chopped

4 large green lettuce leaves, washed and dried

1/3 cup crumbled goat cheese

Directions

In bottom of large bowl, add basil, chicken, brown rice, and mango. Toss well to combine.

Garnish with crumbled goat cheese and serve on top of lettuce leaf.

Creamy Chicken Soup

Ingredients

1 ¹⁄₂ lbs boneless skinless chicken breasts, cut into 2 inch strips

2 teaspoons vegetable oil

2 medium carrots, chopped

2 celery ribs, chopped

1 cup corn, frozen

2 (10 3/4 ounce) cans condensed cream of potato soup, undiluted

1 ¹⁄₂ cups chicken broth

1 teaspoon dill weed

1 cup frozen peas

¹⁄₂ cup skim milk

Directions

In a large skillet over medium high heat, brown chicken in oil. Transfer to a 5 quart slow cooker.

Add the, carrots, celery and corn.

In a small bowl, whisk the soup, broth and dill until blended; stir into slow cooker.

Cover and cook on low for 4 hours or until vegetables are tender.

Stir in peas and cream. Cover and cook 30 minutes longer or until heated through.

PART 2

Chapter 1: What in the world is a thyroid

In this chapter, we will be exploring just what the thyroid is, and its functions in maintaining and keeping your body healthy.

For starters, the word thyroid has its origins dating as far back as the 1690s. Coming from the Greek, thyreoiedes, meaning "shield-shaped". Also referred to as, khondros thyreoiedes, "shield-shaped cartilage". Aptly named, as the thyroid gland is an organ which is often considered to resemble a butterfly, bow tie, or shield shape, at the base of the neck.

The thyroid gland plays an extremely vital role in the way your body uses energy, by releasing hormones that aid in controlling your body's metabolism. The hormones released by the thyroid gland assist in regulating important body functions, including but not limited to:

- Regulation of breathing
- Heart rate
- The central and peripheral nervous systems
- Body weight
- Cycles of menstruation
- The strength of muscles
- Levels of cholesterol
- The temperature of the body

Quite a lot for an organ coming in at only around 2 inches long. This tiny but important gland rests in the front portion of the throat, in front of the trachea, and just below the thyroid cartilage commonly referred to as the Adam's apple. The Adam's apple itself is the largest cartilage of the voice box or larynx.

Owing to the bow tie, butterfly, or shield shape, of the thyroid gland, is a middle connection of thin thyroid tissue, which is known as the isthmus, which is responsible for holding together two lobes on the right and left sides of it. It is not entirely uncommon, however, for someone to be missing the isthmus all-together and instead of having the two lobes of the thyroid gland operating separate from one another.

Now that you are aware of this and may feel a bit more familiar with your own thyroid gland, you may resist trying to see or feel around for it in your neck yourself. Unless the thyroid gland is otherwise afflicted and made to become enlarged, mostly known as a goiter, the thyroid will be unable to be seen, and only just barely able to be felt. It is only when a goiter occurs and the neck is swollen from an enlarged thyroid that it will be at all noticeable either to the eye or to the touch.

The thyroid gland is one of the major players in the endocrine system. The endocrine system includes glands that are responsible for the production and for the secretion of various hormones. The other organs which help make up the endocrine system are the hypothalamus, which is responsible for linking the body's nervous system to the endocrine system via the use of the pituitary gland. The pituitary gland which is responsible for the secretion of hormones, not the blood stream. The pineal gland, which produces the wake/sleep pattern hormone of melatonin. The adrenal glands, which are responsible for the production of a variety of hormones like the steroids cortisol and aldosterone as well as our body's adrenaline. The Pancreas, an organ located in the abdominal region of the body, the primary role of which is the converting of food into fuel for the body's cells. The ovaries and testicles, sex organs of the body. And the parathyroid glands.

Utilizing the iodine content from foods, the thyroid is able to produce and churn out the hormones T3, which stands for triiodothyronine, and the hormone T4, thyroxine.

T3, or triiodothyronine, is merely the active form of the companion hormone thyroxine, or T4. The thyroid gland alone is able to secrete around 20% of our body's T3 into the bloodstream on its own. With the other 80% coming from organs like the liver and the kidneys going through the process of converting thyroxine into its active counterpart.

It is absolutely possible for your body to have far too much of T3 though. When there is an over secretion of

T3 into the blood stream, it is called thyrotoxicosis. This can be due to a number of conditions dealing with the thyroid gland such as overactivity in the thyroid gland, known as hyperthyroidism, caused by such conditions as a benign tumor, the thyroid gland becoming enflamed, or a condition known as graves' disease. The previously mentioned condition of a goiter, in which the neck begins to swell, might be a signal of thyrotoxicosis having occurred. Even more symptoms to have an eye out for in case of hyperthyroidism will be an increase in the appetite, increased regularity of bowel movements, an intolerance to heat, the loss of weight, the menstrual cycle becoming irregulated, a heartbeat becoming increasingly rapid or irregular in rhythm, the thinning or loss of hair, tremors, becoming irritable, overly tired, palpitations, and the eyelids retracting.

It is also possible for your body to be producing too little of the hormone T3. The thyroid gland producing too little of T3 is known commonly as hypothyroidism. It is common for autoimmune diseases to have a strong role in this occurring, an example of which would be the Hashimoto's disease, which causes the immune system to attack the thyroid gland. Certain medications or the intake of too little iodine can also cause hypothyroidism. This can be very serious, especially if a case of hypothyroidism goes unnoticed or untreated during early childhood, or even before birth. With the regulation of hormones being so important, primarily to physical and mental development, not treating hypothyroidism during these crucial times often result in reduced growth for the child, or becoming learning disabled.

The affliction of hypothyroidism is not foreign to adults though. When hypothyroidism occurs in adults they tend to have the functions of their bodies slowed down drastically. The effects of hypothyroidism in an adult have been known to include symptoms such as a growing intolerance to colder temperature, the heart rate of the adult will lower, gaining weight, a reduction in appetite, the ability of memory becomes poorer, fertility will reduce, muscles will become stiff, the adult may become depressed, and tired.

T4, or thyroxine, is the primary hormone that gets secreted from the thyroid gland and into the body's bloodstream. Unlike T3 which is active, thyroxine is in an inactive form and most of it will need to be converted to the active form, triiodothyronine, which is a process that takes place in organs like the kidneys and liver. Undergoing these processes is vital in making sure the body is able to regulate a healthy metabolic rate, control of the body's muscles, development of the brain, develop and maintain bones, and digestive and heart functionality.

As with T3, triiodothyronine, the production and secretion of too much will inevitable result in thyrotoxicosis, while the production and secretion of too little thyroxine, will result in hypothyroidism.

To combat this, the body and thyroid gland have a few tricks vital to the regulation of levels of these hormones in the cells. There is a controlled feedback loop system, involving the hypothalamus in the brain as well as in the thyroid gland and pituitary gland which is in control of the production of both of the hormones thyroxine and triiodothyronine. Thyrotropin-releasing hormones are secreted from the hypothalamus and, in turn, the pituitary gland becomes stimulated into producing thyroid stimulating hormone. A hormone which will stimulate thyroxine and triiodothyronine to be produced and secreted by the thyroid gland.

A feedback loop regulates this production system, to account for the levels of thyroxine and of triiodothyronine. If the levels of either of these thyroid gland hormones begin to increase, they will end up preventing the production and secretion of the thyrotropin-releasing hormone as well as the thyroid stimulating hormone, thus allowing the body to maintain, on it's own, a steady level of the thyroid hormones that it needs.

For all these reasons it is of vital importance that the levels of T3 and T4 being secreted thru-ought the body and its cells never get too high or too low. T3 and T4 are able to reach just about ever cell in the body by utilizing the bloodstream. The rate of work for the cells and metabolism to work is regulated by the hormones T3 and T4. To make sure that levels are never either too high or too low, this is why we have a thyroid gland.

The final hormone that the thyroid gland is responsible for the production of is the hormone calcitonin, CT, or thyrocalcitonin. Within the thyroid gland are what are known as C-cells, or parafollicular cells, which are in charge of the proliferation of this particular hormone. The primary role of calcitonin in the body is to help in the regulation of the levels of phosphate in the blood, and of calcium in the blood. Doing so is to be in opposition of the parathyroid hormone. In short, meaning that what it aims to do is reduce the amount of calcium in the blood stream. The reason for playing this role in the human anatomy game has been a bit of a mystery to science up to this point though, due to the observation of patients showing either very high or even very low levels of the hormone calcitonin, having no adverse effect on them.

The hormone calcitonin has two primary mechanisms by which to aid in the reduction of calcium levels within the human body. It can completely inhibit the activity of the cells in our body which are responsible for breaking down bones, known as osteoclasts. Osteoclasts do this because when bone is broken down, the calcium within the bone being broken down will be released into the body's bloodstream. So by inhibiting the osteoclasts from doing their respective jobs, calcitonin is directly involved in the reduction of the amount of calcium that is getting released into the body's bloodstream. Despite doing this though, the length of time that calcitonin can cause this inhibition has been shown to be quite short. Calcitonin can be an active player in the resorption of calcium into the kidneys, which it does by lower the levels of blood calcium in the body.

Calcitonin has been manufactured in the past and has then been given, in this form, to treat the disease of bone, Paget's disease. Also known as osteitis deformans, Paget's disease is rather common, and is a chronic bone disorder which can cause pain, fractures or deformities of a bone, or show absolutely no symptoms at all. It is however easily able to be controlled and treated with proper early enough diagnosis and treatment.

The manufactured hormone calcitonin has also been given to sufferers of general bone pain, and of hypercalcaemia, which is when the body has an abnormal level of calcium flowing in the bloodstream.

Though because of the introduction of bisphosphonates, which aid in the preventing of the breakdown of bone cells and are drugs also used to help treat osteoporosis, the use of manufactured calcitonin has decreased.

Chapter 2: possible thyroid disorders

In the previous chapter, we began to cover what it is exactly that the thyroid gland gets done and even dabbled a bit into how it does it's job properly. During the last chapter, we mentioned a few of the various thigs which can afflict the thyroid gland, why this may occur in certain circumstances, and what the effects of these afflictions could be. Moving on into chapter two is where we will begin to take a closer look at everything that can go wrong with the thyroid gland. Not just the what, but the why as well. What causes these changes in our thyroid gland to occur, and what to expect to happen when they do occur. The importance of having this knowledge be a part of your thyroid gland arsenal cannot be at all overstated as there is a wide array of severity to both the symptoms and to the results of the ailments that can afflict the thyroid gland and consequently hinder our body's ability to maintain its health properly.

Just as well in this chapter, you can expect to be reading deeper into some of the ailments that may have already been brought up in the previous chapter, such as hyperthyroidism, hypothyroidism, graves disease, goiters, and Hashimoto's disease.

Hyperthyroidism

As briefly discussed in the last chapter, hyperthyroidism is a rather common condition in which there is overactivity in the thyroid gland and begins to produce far too much of the thyroid hormone which would usually be used to regulate the body's metabolic rate. This can be an overproduction of the hormones T3, which is triiodothyronine, T4, which is tetraiodothyronine, or even an overproduction of both of these hormones.

The causes of hyperthyroidism can vary greatly, with the most common reason for it being the aforementioned Grave's disease, which we will go much further into later in the chapter. The basics of Grave's disease are that it is an autoimmune disorder which causes antibodies in the body to stimulate the thyroid gland making it secrete to many of it's hormones. You should tell your regular doctor if any one in your family has ever had Grave's disease as it seems to have a genetic link, being passed down commonly from generation to the next generation. Grave's disease is also known to be more prevalent in women, affecting about 1 percent of the female population, than it is in men.

Another common reason for hyperthyroidism to occur is an excess level of iodine in the body, which is the main ingredient in hormones T3 and T4.

Less common, but still just as relevant to the conversation as causes for hyperthyroidism is thyroiditis which is the inflammation of thyroid gland, which in turn will cause the hormones T3 and T4 to start leaking out of the thyroid gland.

Tumors located on the ovaries or testes have been known links to hyperthyroidism. As well as even tumors, even when benign, located on the thyroid gland, or pituitary gland.

An easily preventable cause of hyperthyroidism which should not be overlooked is the intake of large amounts of T4, or tetraiodothyronine, via the ingestion of a dietary supplement or of a prescribed medication.

When it comes to the symptoms of hyperthyroidism, believe it or not, we had only scratched the surface in the previous chapter and will be going more in-depth here on what you can expect to look out for in order to self-diagnose an issue before going to seek out a professional opinion.

To begin with, in the case of Grave's disease, one of the symptoms can be a bulging of the eyes as if stuck in a stare. Other symptoms to watch out for would be an increase in the appetite, perhaps an increase in nervousness or a sense of restlessness. Muscular weakness, the inability to concentrate on simple tasks, irregularity in the heartbeat, loss of the ability to sleep soundly or for long periods of time, the loss of hair, or noticing that your hair has become thinner or more brittle, can be signs of hyperthyroidism. Thinness of the skin is also common, as well as becoming more irritable, sweating more, or becoming more anxious. In men specifically, the development of breasts can be a sign of hyperthyroidism. And in women, hyperthyroidism has been known to have adverse effects on the regularity of the menstrual cycle.

If you experience any of the prior symptoms, it is, of course, recommended to seek out professional help and diagnosis. However, it is highly recommended that you seek out professional help for the treatment of hyperthyroidism if you begin to experience a sensation of dizziness if you start to notice shortness in your breathing, which will likely come with the increase in heart rate, making it faster and irregular, and any loss of consciousness. Having hyperthyroidism has also been known to be the cause of atrial fibrillations, which are a dangerous arrythmia, commonly responsible for leading to having a stroke, or even to congestive heart failures.

In diagnosing a case of hyperthyroidism, a doctor will likely begin the process by conducting a full and complete medical history, as well as a physical exam. These are commonly conducted as they are helpful in revealing the common signs of loss of weight, how rapid your pulse is, an elevation in pressure of the blood, protrusion of the eyes, or the enlargement of the thyroid gland itself.

It is also reasonable to expect your doctor to conduct a cholesterol test which will be done to check on the levels of cholesterol in your system. This is done because cholesterol levels being low can be an indication that there is an elevation in your metabolic rate, which would mean that your body is burning through your cholesterol far too quickly.

Doctors are also able to conduct tests to measure the levels of T3 and T4 that are in your blood. Thyroid stimulating hormone tests can be done to check the levels of TSH, or thyroid stimulating hormone coursing within your body. TSH stimulates your thyroid gland to produce the hormones the body needs, and if your thyroid gland is producing levels of hormones at a normal rate, or even a rate that is too high, your TSH should come out lower. And a level of TSH that is abnormally low can be an important signifier that you may have hyperthyroidism.

A triglyceride test will be done, because similarly to having low amounts of cholesterol, a low level of triglycerides can be significant of an elevation in your metabolic rate. A thyroid scan or uptake will allow a doctor to see if your thyroid gland is being overactive. It will actually get even more particular, and let a doctor be able to see if it is the entire thyroid gland which is acting up or just a particular area of the thyroid gland.

Ultrasounds have been known to be utilized, as they will allow a doctor to observe entirely, the size of the thyroid gland, as well as any masses that may be within the thyroid gland. It is the use of the ultrasound which will also be able to let the doctor know if the mass inside the thyroid gland is cystic, or if it is solid. Just as well a CT, Computed Tomography, or MRI, Magnetic Resonance Imaging, scan can be performed to show if the condition is being caused by a tumor being present on the pituitary gland.

Treatment of hyperthyroidism also comes in varieties and may be dependent on the cause of the hyperthyroidism. Perhaps the most common treatment comes in the form of medication. Generally an antithyroid medication like methimazole, also known as Tapazole, which will cause the thyroid gland to halt the production and secretion of hormones altogether.

According to the American Thyroid Association, around 70 percent of U.S. adults who undergo treatment for hyperthyroidism will receive a form of treatment called radioactive iodine. Radioactive iodine is essentially able to completely and effectively destroy the cells that would otherwise be producing hormones. Radioactive iodine, or RAI, in the form of a liquid or a pill, will be ingested by way of the mouth, and is safe to use on an individual who has had any allergic reaction to an X-ray contrast agent or to seafood, because essentially the reaction comes from the compound which contains iodine, and not from the iodine itself. The iodine, in an iodide form, is actually split into two forms or radioactive iodine, known as I-123, which is harmless to thyroid gland cells, and I-131, which is responsible for the destruction of thyroid gland cells. The radiation which is emitted by both of these forms of the iodine are able to be detected from outside of the patient, which will help the doctor to gain any information needed the thyroid glands functionality, and take any pictures needed of the size thyroid glands tissues, as well as their location in the body. This treatment is not without its side effects though, which generally tend to come in the presence of dryness of the mouth, soreness of the eyes and in the throat, and has also been known to effect changes in taste. You may also be required, if undergoing this treatment, to take precautions for a short time which will prevent the spread of radiation to others.

Surgery is yet another common form of treatment for hyperthyroidism. In this case, it is entirely possible that a section of your thyroid gland will be removed, though entire thyroid glands have also been removed in this procedure. This is followed up with taking thyroid hormone supplements which will help in the prevention of hypothyroidism, which is what happens when there is the occurrence of underactivity in the thyroid gland, causing it to produce and secrete too little of the intended hormones. Beta-blockers may also be taken, such as something like propranolol to help control a rapid pulse, sweating, any anxiety that may crop up, and higher blood pressure. It is reported that most people respond very well to this form of treatment.

If you would like to improve any symptoms, or even take action to prevent symptoms from occurring, you are not left without options. You can work along with your doctor, or a dietician, to help create a healthy guideline for diet, exercise, and any nutritional supplementation. Proper diet intake, with a stronger focus on getting calcium and sodium, can be crucially important in the prevention of hyperthyroidism. Osteoporosis is a common result of hyperthyroidism as it can make your bones become thin, weak, and very brittle. To strengthen the bones after treatment for hyperthyroidism, it is recommended to take calcium supplements and vitamin D. To get an idea of how much vitamin D you should be taking post-surgery, you can talk to your doctor for a recommendation.

Moving on from treatment, it is not unusual for a doctor to recommend their patients to an endocrinologist, who will be more specialized in the treatment of systems dealing with bodily hormones. You'll want to avoid stress at this stage as it can cause thyroid storm, which happens when a large amount of thyroid hormone gets released, resulting in a horrible and sudden worsening of any prior symptoms. Proper treatment is both recommended and effective at the prevention of thyroid storm, as well as other complications such as thyrotoxicosis.

In the long-term, the outlook for something like hyperthyroidism is dependent heavily on what is causing it. Some of the causes of hyperthyroidism can go away without ever seeking treatment. Whereas a more serious cause like Graves' disease is not to be taken lightly, as it will get much worse if it goes without treatment, and the complications due to Graves' disease are often life-threatening and will have an affect on your quality of life long-term. These are easy enough to subdue with proper care and an early diagnosis and treatment.

Hypothyroidism

Though we went over a little about hypothyroidism in chapter 1, it is important to take a closer look at the disorder, to gain a better idea of its symptoms, and proper treatment and care for it.

When the body is not producing enough of the thyroid hormones that it needs, this is what is known as hypothyroidism having occurred. This will cause the general functions of your body to become slowed down, as the thyroid gland is responsible for producing and secreting hormones which will provide energy to nearly every other portion of your body. Though this affliction can come to task at any age, it is more common for an underactive thyroid gland to be noticed in adults over the age of 60, as well as being more prevalent in women. A diagnosis of hypothyroidism is nothing to get too worked up about, fortunately, as treatment of hypothyroidism has been known to be quite effective, as well as being very simple and very safe.

Though the symptoms of having an underactive thyroid gland can vary from person to person, there is enough overlap in the symptoms for us to help lay out what to look out for. It is important to note, however, that there can be difficulty in pin-pointing that a symptom is that of hypothyroidism and that the severity of the condition itself plays a large role in which signs or symptoms will appear, as well as when they may make an appearance.

It is not at all uncommon for most people to experience the symptoms of this condition arriving in a slow progression over many years. The thyroid gland will grow ever slower and slower, which will only then allow the symptoms to be better identifiable. The trouble can become that many of the symptoms come with general aging, so if you suspect there is more to the picture, and that hypothyroidism is at play, it is important to go see a doctor. An example of some early symptoms which also come naturally with age are the symptomatic fatigue and gaining of weight.

If hypothyroidism does occur, however, other symptoms to keep an eye out for will be an uptick in depression, constipation, or muscle weakness. It is also common to begin becoming more sensitive to the cold, for the skin to become dry, and a reduction in sweating. Your heart rate will generally become slower, blood cholesterol may elevate, and joints may become stiff or experience more pain. It is also possible for memory to start becoming impaired, hair may thin or become dry. Your voice may become hoarse, muscles will stiffen and experience soreness, your face will become puffy and sensitive. In women, hypothyroidism as been known to negatively affect menstrual changes and cause difficulty in fertility.

When it comes to the causes of hypothyroidism, an autoimmune disease is fairly common to be the culprit at work. The body is designed in such a way that your immune system generally will protect the body's cells against any invading bacteria and virus. Therefore, when an unknown virus or bacteria enters the body, it is the immune system which will respond by sending out what are known as fighter cells, to destroy the foreign invading virus or bacteria.

However, it is not impossible for your body to begin confusing what are the healthy and normal cells, with the invading cells. This is what is then called an autoimmune response to the cells. And if this autoimmune response does not get properly treated, or if it is not properly regulated, it is your own immune system which will start to attack your healthy body tissues. Medically, this has been known to cause quite serious issues, which include hypothyroidism.

Hashimoto's disease, which we have mentioned before, is one such autoimmune condition that can occur, and it is the most common among the causes of having an underactive thyroid gland. The disease literally will attack the thyroid gland which will cause chronic thyroid inflammation, which, in turn, will reduce the functionality of the thyroid gland. As with Graves' disorder having links between generations, it is not at all uncommon to find that multiple members of a family have this same condition as well.

Hypothyroidism can even become an occurrence as a result of treatment for hyperthyroidism, which has the aim of lowering your thyroid hormone. It is not uncommon for the treatment to result in keeping the thyroid hormone too low, which then becomes hypothyroidism, which has been a known result of the radioactive iodine treatment for hyperthyroidism.

The surgical removal of the thyroid gland is yet another known cause of the occurrence of hypothyroidism. The entirety of the thyroid gland will be removed in the case of thyroid problems cropping up, which will affect the body's ability to produce thyroid hormone, and cause hypothyroidism. In this instance, you will typically be recommended to take thyroid medication for the rest of your life. In the case that it is only a smaller portion of the thyroid gland which is removed, it is possible for the thyroid gland to still be able to produce and secrete a healthy amount of hormones. In which case it will take a test of the blood to determine how much medication you will need.

It is possible for radiation therapy to be the cause if you have come down with hypothyroidism. A diagnosis of leukemia, neck cancer, or lymphoma will likely mean you have had to undergo a form of radiation therapy, which very nearly almost leads to the occurrence of hypothyroidism.

Just as possible, is a medication you may be taking to lower thyroid gland hormone production, to be the cause of hypothyroidism. Medications such as these are commonly used in the treatment of certain psychological diseases, and even have been known to be used in treating heart disease and cancer.

When it comes down the diagnosing of hypothyroidism, there are two primary methods which have been favored and work to best identify when it has occurred. The first being a strict medical evaluation, much like in the case of checking for hyperthyroidism. The doctor will give you a very thorough exam physically, as well as making sure to go over your medical history. Hypothyroidism has a couple physical signs which the doctor will be checking for primarily such as the dryness of the skin, how slow or quick your reflexes are, any swelling of the neck, and the rate of your heart beat. It is at this time that a doctor will also likely ask you to report any of the other symptoms listed earlier that you may have experienced, such as the depression, any fatigue, if you have been constipated, and a sensation of being more sensitive to the cold. It is also at this point it will be most helpful for you to let the doctor know of any thyroid conditions which have existed in your family.

To reliably get an idea of the existence of hypothyroidism in the body, it is required to conduct blood tests. It is only by this method that anyone will be able to tell and get a look at a measure of your body's thyroid-stimulating hormone levels, done by utilizing a thyroid-stimulating hormone test to see how much of the thyroid-stimulating hormone your pituitary gland is or is not creating. In the case that your thyroid gland is not producing enough of the hormone, the pituitary gland will respond to this by boosting the thyroid-stimulating hormone it produces in order to increase thyroid hormone production. If it turns out you have hypothyroidism, the levels of thyroid-stimulating hormone in your body will be increased, because your body is responding by making an attempt at stimulating more thyroid gland hormone activity. If hyperthyroidism is what ails you, the levels of the thyroid-stimulating hormone in your body will as having decreased, because in this case, your body has begun the process of attempting to halt the function of excessive production of the thyroid glands hormones.

Another useful method in the detection and diagnosis of hypothyroidism is to test the levels of T4 in the body, being produced by your thyroid gland, as T4 is produced directly by the thyroid gland. When they are used in conjunction with one another, a test of T4 levels and the thyroid-stimulating hormone test are very helpful in coming up with an evaluation of thyroid gland functionality. In general, if you the levels of thyroid-stimulating hormone in your body has increased, while the level of the hormone T4 has decreased, you much more than likely have hypothyroidism. Though, due to the sheer amount of conditions that can have such a negative impact on the thyroid gland, it could very well end up being necessary to conduct even more tests of the thyroid glands function I order to properly diagnose the issue.

Though it is true that for many people who have thyroid conditions, that the right amount of the proper medication will assist in the alleviation of their symptoms, you will have hypothyroidism for the rest of your life if you get it.

To get the best of hypothyroidism it is most commonly treated the best with the use of levothyroxine, also known as Levothroid or Levoxyl, which is T4 put into a synthetic form that is responsible for copying the action the thyroid hormone would regularly take if it were being produced as normal by your body. The idea behind doing this is that the medication will cause a return to the proper levels of the thyroid hormone in your blood. Once a restoration of the thyroid hormone level has occurred, many of the symptoms that come along with having hypothyroidism, will at the very least become much easier to manage, and at best the hypothyroidism symptoms will disappear altogether. It is important to expect it to take several weeks, following treatment, before relief sets in, and you start to feel a return to normalcy. There will also very likely be follow up appointments for testing your blood, which the doctor will recommend in order to keep a solid eye on your progress into recovery. Chances are that you will also receive some medication or other recommended methods to aid you in your recovery, be sure to speak with your doctor about the dosage you should be taking and to come up with a solid plan, that will most benefit you, for recovering in a timely fashion.

It is the case that many people who end up with hypothyroidism medicate for it, for the rest of their lives. Despite this, the dosage you will be taking thru ought that time is likely to go through changes. To better get an idea of how these dosages should be changing over time, it is best to get a check up on your thyroid-stimulation hormone levels every year. In this way, your doctor will be able to more properly adjust the amount you should be taking, or not taking, based on the blood levels indicated by the thyroid-stimulating hormone tests. Only by doing this regularly, will you and your doctor be able to achieve the recovery program that works best for you.

Plans and programs for this achievement may include medications and other hormone supplementation.

Once again, synthetic versions of the hormone you need may be used, as they are a widely used and viable practice to aid in the recovery of hypothyroidism. The synthetic version of the hormone T3 is liothyronine, and T4 in its synthetic medication form is called levothyroxine, both of which act as suitable substitutes for their corresponding hormone.

If it was a deficiency in your iodine intake which caused your specific occurrence of hypothyroidism, it is likely that your doctor will recommend a supplementary form of iodine. Keep in mind to ask your doctor, and get the proper testing before taking anything, but selenium and magnesium supplements have been known to aid heavily in the treatment of hypothyroidism.

The golden ticket to any recovery or treatment is usually diet, and in the case of hypothyroidism, there is no exception. Though this is the case, and diet can be incredibly beneficial in your recovery and treatment, do not expect a change in your diet, doctor recommended or otherwise, to replace the need for a prescribed medication. Foods that are rich in selenium or magnesium such as nuts and seeds like the Brazil nut and sunflower seeds have been shown to be very beneficial additions to any diet to aid in the treatment of hypothyroidism.

Balance in your diet will play an especially important role, as the thyroid gland requires particular amounts of iodine in order to properly reach full functionality. There are foods such as whole grains, vegetables, fruits, and lean meats which can handily accomplish this without the need for iodine supplementation.

And of course, diet is only the beginning, exercise as well comes in as an important slice of the treatment and recovery pie. The muscle and joint pain that coincides with hypothyroidism will more often than not leave one to feel extreme fatigue and depression, both of which can be helped by creating and sticking to a regular work out regime. Though no exercise should be discounted, unless specifically told to avoid certain activities by your doctor, there are certain ones which will prove more beneficial than others for treating the symptoms of hypothyroidism. Low impact workouts such as swimming, riding a bike, doing Pilates or yoga, or even a good brisk walk, have been known to be very helpful low impact work outs that are helpful and easy to work in to a daily routine.

The building up of muscle mass by strength training, lifting weights, sit ups, pushups, and pull-ups, help reduce the lethargic feeling of sluggishness that comes along with hypothyroidism. The increase in muscle mass will result in an increase in the rate of your metabolism, which will simultaneously assist in decreasing any weight gain that the hypothyroidism may have caused.

And finally doing training that is primarily cardiovascular. As stated earlier, hypothyroidism is one of the ailments that can correlate with a heightened risk of having a cardiac arrythmia, or irregularity of the heartbeat. By taking steps to be more mindful of your cardiovascular health, exercising on a regular basis or schedule, will help in protecting your heart.

There are also alternative treatments which exist to help in taking care of hypothyroidism, such as animal extracts that contain the thyroid hormone. These extracts are made available from pigs because they contain both the thyroid hormone T4 and thyroid hormone T3. It is uncommon for these to be recommended, however, as they have not shown to be reliable in how to dose, as well as not being more effective than the typically recommended medications. It is also popular to find some glandular extracts in stores that are health food based. The risk that comes along with them is that the U.S. Food and Drug Administration plays no role in the monitoring or the regulation of these extracts. This has historically brought the guarantee of their pureness, legitimacy, and even their potency into question. If you decide to use these products, you do so at your own risk, but still be sure to inform your doctor so that they can adjust accordingly to your treatment.

You can go above and beyond in regards to hypothyroidism treatment, yet still deal with issues or complications that are longer lasting because of this harsh fluctuation to your body. Luckily there have been methods developed and used which will help to lessen the burden of hypothyroidisms effects on your life moving forward.

In the beginning, fatigue can feel like a lot to deal with, especially when associated with depression. These feelings can creep through even if you are taking proper dosages of your medication. It is of utmost importance that you get a good quality sleep every night to ease your treatment and recovery. A good, healthy diet, as well as the relief of stress through activities such as meditation, Pilates, and yoga, are effective strategies when it comes to combating lower energy levels.

It is also vitally important to recognize the difficulty of having a medical condition that is chronic, especially in the case of something like hypothyroidism, which comes along with its own mixed bag of other concerns to your overall health. Being able to talk about, or express, the experience of going through this will help. There are resources out there for support groups of other people who live with the effects of hypothyroidism, you can find a therapist to talk to, perhaps a close friend or loved one. Anyone who will be able to enable you to discuss your experience with openness and with honesty. You may even be able to receive a recommendation for meetings of people with hypothyroidism, from an education office at your local hospital. Connecting and communicating with others who can empathize with what you are going through could end up being an enormous aid in your recovery and life with hypothyroidism.

Important as well is making sure you monitor yourself for other health conditions that could arise. As we went over earlier, the main cause for hypothyroidism is an autoimmune disease. Just as well, links with hypothyroidism have also been found in conditions such as diabetes, having pituitary issues, having your sleep obstructed by sleep apnea, and lupus.

Just as with fatigue, depression is a common symptom and side effect of going through and living with hypothyroidism and should be watched closely. The thyroid glands hormone levels lower, the function of your body begins to slow down, and before you may realize it you are living with a depression that was not there before. It is vital to know what to look out for, and not just what, but also how to look after yourself while dealing with this.

Depression as a symptom can make hypothyroidism difficult to diagnose as there are many who may only experience difficulties or changes in mood as a symptom. It is for this reason, that instead of having a doctor check only your brain when checking for depression, it can also be important to ask them to check for signs of you having an underactive thyroid. Aside from the changes in mood, there are a few other similarities that exist in both having depression as well as hypothyroidism such as, gaining weight, finding it difficult to maintain concentration, feelings of daily fatigue, which coincide with a reduced desire and satisfaction with daily life, and hypothyroidism or depression could both effect your ability to sleep well.

Not all of their symptoms overlap so nicely though, both have their conditions which differentiate one from the other. In the case of hypothyroidism there are, of course, some physical signs such as the dryness of the skin, or the thinning and loss of hair. There is also the tendency to become constipated and the increase in levels of cholesterol. These symptoms would be atypical if depression alone was the issue.

If you have hypothyroidism and it is the cause of your depression, then the correct treatment and care of the hypothyroidism should be just the remedy needed in order to treat your depression as well. If the hypothyroidism passes and depression remains, it may be important to talk to your doctor about receiving further help and a change in medication.

Along with depression being a symptom of hypothyroidism, it has recently been found, through studies, that around 60 percent or so of people who get hypothyroidism tend to also exhibit having anxiety as well. Studies are ongoing and are still growing in scope and size, though it would still be in your best interest to discuss all possibilities and symptoms with your doctor in order to more thoroughly and best tackle the treatment of hypothyroidism.

It cannot be stressed enough, how much of your body is under the affects and influence of your thyroid gland working properly to produce and secrete the correct levels of hormones. For this reason, when a woman gets hypothyroidism and simultaneously desires to get pregnant, she will be faced with her own subset of challenges to come. Have a low thyroid gland function during a pregnancy can cause a number of conflicts including various birth defects, have a still-birth or miscarriage, as well as anemia or a low birth weight. It is not uncommon for a woman with thyroid problems to have a perfectly healthy pregnancy, but to make sure that you reach this outcome it is important to do things such as eating well, keeping yourself informed about current and effective medicines, as well as talking to your doctor about testing.

Though testing may result in changes to your dosage or medication, it is also for this reason that it is important to make sure you are not deviating from the medications provided and the dosage your doctor has recommended.

Considering the thyroid issues adds on even more importance to the need for eating healthy while pregnant. Make sure that you are getting the proper amount of vitamins, minerals, and nutrients and consider taking multivitamins as well to supplement this.

It is not impossible to develop a thyroid issue such as hypothyroidism while pregnant. In fact, for every 1,000 pregnancies, this tends to occur in every 3 out of 5 women. It is important for doctors to routinely check thyroid levels during your pregnancy, as some will do, to make sure your thyroid levels aren't becoming to high or low. If they end up being higher or lower than they ought to be, it is likely that your doctor will recommend you starting treatment. Even some women who have never before had any thyroid issues may develop them once the baby is born, which is known as postpartum thyroiditis, and also tends to resolve itself after a year in around 80 percent of the women it shows up in. It is only the other 20 percent of women who will have this happen and then go on to require the long term treatment.

When hypothyroidism takes place, and the functions of the body slow down, it is quite typical for people to become prone to gaining weight, which is very likely due to what happens to the bodies ability to burn energy, which is that the efficiency to do so slows down as well. This change in the body will typically cause someone who has hypothyroidism to gain anywhere from 5 to 10 pounds in general, making the weight that is gained not entirely drastic, but someone could still find it quite alarming. It is very possible then, that once the hypothyroidism has been treated, that any weight gained will then be easily lost. If this does not occur, a simple change in diet, and adding regular exercise to your routine should aid in handily losing the weight, as your ability to manage weight will go back to normalcy, with the return to proper levels in your thyroid hormones.

Hypothyroidism is a common occurrence; therefore it is also commonly treated without issue. Hypothyroidism has been found to occur in around 4.6 percent of the American population that are 12 and older. Which comes out to about 10 million or so people who go on to live long healthy lives with the condition, and you may never even realize it. It is far more prevalent in people who are over the age of 60, and in women about 1 in 5 of them are likely to experience hypothyroidism by the time they have reached 60 years of age. One of the causes is Hashimoto's disease which happens to appear more in women who have reached middle-age, though it can absolutely show up in children and men. As Hashimoto's disease is hereditary, it is likely that if you get it, you did so from a relative, and have an increased chance then of passing it on down to your children.

It is important to keep an eye on your body, your health, and your thyroid gland as you get older. If, as the years go by, you begin to notice any of the changes gone over in this chapter so far, it is vital that you see a doctor in an attempt to get a proper diagnosis and seek treatment as soon as possible.

Hashimoto's Disease

Hashimoto's disease is an autoimmune disease which can be very destructive to your thyroid gland, and thereby your thyroid glands ability to function properly. Hashimoto's disease is also known as chronic autoimmune lymphocytic thyroiditis and is the most common cause of having an underactive thyroid gland, hypothyroidism, in the United States.

As an autoimmune disorder, Hashimoto's disease is one of many conditions that will be the cause of your body's white blood cells and your body's antibodies becoming confused and starting to attack the cells that make up the thyroid gland. What makes this happen precisely is still somewhat of a mystery to doctors, even still it is believed by some that factors of genetics may be involved.

With the cause of Hashimoto's disease being unknown, it is difficult to precisely put a finger on what puts a person at risk for having or contracting the disease. There are still, however, just a few factors that doctors are aware of which could signify being at risk for the disease. In the case of Hashimoto's disease, in particular, women happen to be seven times more likely to contract than men, and especially for women who have been pregnant before. Having a history of autoimmune diseases in the family is another factor that could mean you are at higher risk of having Hashimoto's at some point in your life, especially if the autoimmune diseases include Graves' disease, lupus, rheumatoid arthritis, if there is a history of Sjogren's syndrome in your family, or a history of type 1 diabetes, Addison's disease, and vitiligo. If it is the case that these autoimmune diseases are present in your family line or may have been based on symptoms of Hashimoto's disease, get together and discuss the possibility with your doctor, then make sure to get tested for the disease.

Hashimoto's disease is interesting in that the symptoms of it, are not symptomatic of Hashimoto's disease alone, in fact, they are similar to having the symptoms of an underactive thyroid gland, or hypothyroidism. Some signs to watch out for that your thyroid gland is not working properly to produce proper thyroid hormones, and that you may have Hashimoto's disease are your skin becoming dry and pale, constipation, if your voice becomes hoarse, you become depressed and start to feel sluggish or fatigued. High levels of cholesterol, a thinning of the hair, muscle weakness in the lower body, and intolerance to the cold may also be signs of hypothyroidism as a result of Hashimoto's disease. In women, it can also cause issues with fertility. Hashimoto's can exist inside of your body for many years before you begin to show any signs or symptoms, and during that time, it may progress while showing no signs of damage to the thyroid gland. Some with Hashimoto's disease end up with a goiter, an enlarging of the thyroid gland which causes the front of the neck to swell. Though generally painless, it is common for a goiter to make the act of swallowing difficult and for it to simulate a feeling of fullness in the throat.

Owing to it's difficulty to diagnose, your doctor may not suspect Hashimoto's of being prevalent until observing symptoms having hypothyroidism. In which case they will need to conduct a blood test designed to check the thyroid-stimulating hormone, or TSH, levels in your body. It is a relatively common and safe test, which is also an accurate way to check to see if you have Hashimoto's disease. Levels of thyroid-stimulating hormone are higher when the activity of the thyroid glad is lower because your body starts working harder to stimulate the production of more thyroid hormones to secrete from the thyroid gland. There are also blood tests that your doctor may conduct if they feel the need to check further for the levels of antibodies, cholesterol, and other thyroid hormones, T3 and T4, in your blood. Testing for all of these can help immensely in pinning down a diagnosis of Hashimoto's disease.

Unless your thyroid gland is functioning normally, in which case your doctor may still recommend regular checkups to monitor you for any changes, it is very likely that the need for treatment of Hashimoto's disease will be required.

The improper production of enough hormones in your body by your thyroid gland will likely result in the need to take medication. In the case of having to take this medication, it is also likely that you will be prescribed on it, though dose will vary, for the rest of your life. The effective drug most commonly prescribed is levothyroxine which is the hormone thyroxine, or T4, made synthetically, and which will successfully replace the missing hormone in your blood. The synthetic hormone drug levothyroxine tends not to have any noticeable side effects, and regular use has been known to frequently return the hormone levels of the body back to normal, restoring proper function of the thyroid gland. When this happens, all other symptoms of Hashimoto's disease and hypothyroidism generally tend to disappear altogether, though it is likely that your doctor will still recommend that you still get regular testing done so that your hormone levels can be consistently monitored to prevent something like hypothyroidism from becoming a problem again moving forward. Getting the regular testing allows the doctor to adjust the dosage of your medication as necessary if at all necessary.

It is important to consider before going on levothyroxine, that there are supplements and medications which will have an effect on your body's ability to absorb the drug. As such, make sure you have a discussion about this with your doctor if you are taking any other medications, especially if they include iron or calcium supplements, or estrogen. Some medications for cholesterol have been known to cause an issue, as well as proton pump inhibitors which are used as a treatment for acid reflux.

Though these have been known to cause an issue, there is what could be an easy work around of simply changing what time of the day you take your other medicines in conjunction with the doctor recommended thyroid medicine. It is also possible that certain foods could end up being involved in the efficacy of your thyroid medicine. It is best to discuss all of this with your doctor to come up with an efficient way for you to take your thyroid medicine, based on your dietary needs.

The severity of complications due to leaving Hashimoto's untreated varies and are not worth the risk if you ever contract, or if you have it. They go far beyond just hypothyroidism and include heart problems that an include total failure of the heart. It is not unusual for anemia to be a result of leaving Hashimoto's disease unattended. Depression and a decrease in libido are common, as well as higher levels of cholesterol in the blood and experiencing a sense of confusion or loss of consciousness.

Hashimoto's disease has also been the culprit responsible for complications during a woman's pregnancy cycle. It is far more likely, that if you carry out a pregnancy while having untreated Hashimoto's disease, that you may be putting your child at higher risk of being born with defects of their kidneys, their heart, and even their brains.

These complications can be limited by talking to your doctor during the pregnancy and keeping on top of monitoring your thyroid glands hormone levels with the proper blood testing. If you are a pregnant woman and have thyroid issues, such preventative measures could mean a severe change in the life and health of your child. However, if you have not had any known disorders with your thyroid or hormone levels, it is not recommended that you get regular or constant screening done during the pregnancy.

Graves' Disease

Another autoimmune disorder, Graves' disease is responsible for causing your thyroid gland too create too much of the thyroid hormones in your body. When this happens it is a condition referred to commonly as hyperthyroidism. Graves' disease, is named such for the man who discovered it, an Irish physician named Robert J. Graves, and is regarded as one of the most common forms hyperthyroidism takes, having an effect on around 1 out of every 200 people.

When Graves' disease occurs in the body, it will cause your immune system to begin creating antibodies that are known as thyroid-stimulating immunoglobulins, that attach themselves to the body's usually healthy cells of the thyroid gland. By doing this they end up causing the thyroid gland to produce and secrete more of the thyroid hormones than it is meant to for your body. The hormones that are produced by the thyroid gland go on to affect a great number of your body's functions including its temperature, the function of the nervous system, the development of the brain, and the list goes on. For this reason, hyperthyroidism can end up having a negatively driven affect on not just all of those functions, but when left untreated can also cause the loss of weight and mental and physical fatigue. Hyperthyroidism has also been found to be responsible for such things as depression and emotional liability where the individual will uncontrollably cry or laugh or put on other manic emotional displays.

Due to the role that Graves' disease can invariably play on the appearance of hyperthyroidism in the body, it is no surprise that the two would contain a sharing of many of the same symptoms. These symptoms include tremors especially of the hands, a loss of weight, tachycardia, which is the rapidity in the rate of the heart, becoming intolerant to heat or warmth, fatigue, nervousness and irritability, the swelling of the front of the neck, due to the enlargement of the thyroid gland, known as a goiter, an increase in the frequency of having bowel movements, as well as diarrhea, weakness of the muscles, and having it become difficult to get a good full night's worth of sleep. Among the people who experience having Graves' disease, it is only a small percentage who will experience the skin thickening around their shin area and become reddened, an affliction which is known as Graves' dermopathy.

Another common symptom of Graves' disease which one may go through while experiencing the condition, is what is called Graves' ophthalmopathy. Graves' ophthalmopathy is what occurs when the eyes of the afflicted individual appear to be enlarged, which is a result of the eyelids retracting. When Graves' ophthalmopathy happens, it is entirely possible that your eyes may begin to bulge outwards from your eye sockets. Estimates say that as much as 30 percent of the people who end up developing Graves' disease will observe at least a mild case of what is known as Graves' ophthalmopathy and that for up to 5 percent of the people will instead experience an extreme case of the eye bulging.

Because of autoimmune diseases such as Graves' disease, the immune system will begin to fight against what are the healthy cells and healthy tissues of the body. Normally, your immune system is producing proteins which are known as antibodies, which are responsible for fighting against foreign invaders to your body, the likes of harmful viruses and bacteria. The antibodies produced this way are formed especially with the duty of targeting a specific invader to the host. When it comes to the effect of Graves' disease on the body, your immune system begins to mistake healthy thyroid cells as these foreign harmful cells and produces the thyroid-stimulating immunoglobulins which then mistakenly go off to attack what are your healthy thyroid cells.

Scientists and doctors alike, are aware that it is indeed possible for a person to have inherited the ability for their body to make antibodies which then go against their own healthy cells, yet they have made no determination that such an occurrence is what is the cause for Graves' disease, or who will end up developing Graves' disease.

Despite that though, there are experts who believe that they have been able to button down on some factors which may increase ones risk for the development of graves disease which includes its tendency to be hereditary. So be sure to discuss family medical history with your doctor and talk about whether or not there are family members who have, or who ay have had Graves' disease. It is also believed by these experts that stress, gender, and someone's age may be some of the facets that end up putting someone at higher risk of getting Graves' disease. It is typical for the disease to be found in people who are younger than the age of 40, and it has been more prevalent, about seven to eight times so, in women rather than men.

Having had, or having still, another autoimmune disease is yet another factor that will increase your risk of ever getting Graves' disease. Examples of such autoimmune diseases are having Crohn's disease, rheumatoid arthritis, and diabetes mellitus, among others.

For the diagnosing of Graves' disease, when it is suspected, it is not unheard of for your doctor to request lab tests. The use of your families medical history as well, especially if there is a case of someone in your family having had Graves' disease, will be able to help act as a basis for your doctor to zero in on diagnosing whether you have Graves' disease as well or not. This is something that thyroid gland blood tests will be needed for in order to confirm. Your doctor may request that these tests and others may be handled by a specialist expert in diseases which are related to the body's hormones, known as an endocrinologist, in order to help get the diagnosis of Graves' disease. Other tests which your doctor may request are full bloodwork tests, a thyroid gland scan, an uptake test utilizing radioactive iodine, a test for levels of TSH, or thyroid stimulating hormone, and a TSI test, which is the thyroid-stimulating immunoglobulins.

By combining the efforts of the endocrinologist, as well as the array of tests, it is more possible for your doctor to determine if you do indeed have and need treatment for Graves' disease specifically, or if another thyroid disorder is what is at work, and thus requires its own specific form of treatment.

There are a number of options available for treatment when someone is diagnosed as having Graves' disease. These are generally the taking of anti-thyroid drugs, therapy in the form of RAI, or radioactive iodine, and getting thyroid gland surgery. It is not abnormal for a doctor, in the case of Graves' disease, to recommend, all, two, or just one of the treatments for the afflicted.

When it comes to treatment via anti-thyroid drugs, you will typically be taking medications such as methimazole, which is taken orally as a tablet and works by putting a stop to the thyroid gland producing and secreting too much thyroid hormone, and propylthiouracil, which is also taken orally and generally used as a back up if a drug like methimazole did not end up working well enough. The use of beta-blockers is also recommended on occasion as they are used in assistance of reducing the effects of symptoms until another treatment method can start working.

It is radioactive iodine treatment, or RAI, which is among the most common treatments suggested to those suffering of Graves' disease. It is required, during this treatment, that the individual seeking treatment take specified doses of radioactive iodine-131, the purpose of which is to destroy thyroid cells. The radioactive iodine-131 will be ingested orally, in small amounts, via pill. Be sure to discuss with your doctor and risks or precautions that come with this treatment.

The less frequent option for treatment is the thyroid surgery. This treatment will tend to be a last resort if the other options have not worked to full capacity, if there is a reason to be suspect of thyroid cancer being present, or if the patient is a pregnant woman who is unable to take any of the regularly prescribed anti-thyroid drugs.

In the case of surgery being necessary, it is not uncommon the doctor to issue the removal of your thyroid gland completely, in the interest of preventing the return of the hyperthyroidism. In which case, thyroid hormone replacement surgery will be necessary on a regular basis. Talk to your doctor about the possible side effects of choosing to go through with surgery, as well as generally what to expect moving forward.

Goiter

A goiter, goitre, thyroid cyst, or Plummer's disease, is a general term used for when there is an observable enlargement of the thyroid gland, usually resulting in a noticeable swelling of the front of the neck. Treatment for a goiter can be handled in a variety of ways, and the treatment method is dependent on the goiters location, the length of its presence, and how exactly it is affecting the thyroid glands performance.

Though usually unable to be seen or even felt, the thyroid gland generally tends to become detectable by touch and even perceptible to the eye when there is a goiter present. An expanse of the thyroid gland, or goiter, can be the cause of the whole thyroid gland expanding, which is known as a "smooth goiter", or just a part of the thyroid gland expanding, which is also called a "cystic" or "nodular" goiter. A goiter is not a sure symptom of having an active thyroid, known as hyperthyroidism, or underactive thyroid, known as hypothyroidism, and, in fact, the majority of people who have a goiter, retain a perfectly normal use of their thyroid gland.

A number of reasons exist for the existence of a goiter. Among these are included a deficiency in your levels of iodine. Iodine may be a trace element, but it is far from trivial. It assists in helping the thyroid gland in maintaining proper functionality and making the thyroid glands hormones. There are two primary hormones which are produced and secreted by the thyroid gland, these are T4 or thyroxine, and T3, also known as triiodothyronine. The approximate number of people who have iodine deficiency comes out to about 2.2 billion and it is estimated that around 29 percent of the worlds total population live in an area that is considered to be deficient in iodine. It is reported that people in the U.K. have proper levels of iodine as a part of their regular diet. If you are keeping your eye out for food sources that are a good source of iodine, there are salts that have iodine supplements, as well, non-organic milk is plentiful with iodine.

Thyroiditis is anther well known cause of goiter. Thyroiditis is more commonly referred to as when the thyroid gland has become inflamed. Around the world, the most common reason for thyroiditis occurring is Hashimoto's disease, or Hashimoto's thyroiditis, which is an autoimmune disease that causes the bodies antibodies to start to become confused and begin attacking healthy cells of the thyroid gland. Hashimoto's disease is not the only cause of the thyroiditis condition though, it could also stem from viral infection, and has been known to occur just after or during pregnancy.

A goiter has also been known to occur due to Graves' disease, another autoimmune disease, this one causing the immune systems antibodies attacks on thyroid cells to make the thyroid gland overactive, resulting in hyperthyroidism. It is this hyperthyroidism, or over activity of the thyroid glands capacity for producing and secreting hormones, which is the cause of the swelling of the thyroid gland.

If there are benign growths on the thyroid gland, they have been known to cause a goiter, most commonly known for doing this is a follicular adenoma, which can be a firm or rubbery tumor surrounded by a fibrous capsule.

External factors that may be the cause of goiter are known as goitrogens. Included among what would be considered a goitrogen are medicines such as the mental health drug lithium, and cabbage type vegetables. Ingestion in the excess of these vegetables, which include cassava or kelp, will likely result in the growth formation of a goiter.

There are physiological demands put on the body during pregnancy and during puberty which have been known to be at the root of a goiter. And as with other causes like Graves' disease and Hashimoto's disease, there is a strong likelihood of inherited genetic reasons that one may at some point experience goiter.

Due to the varying reasons for the existence of goiter, there are also a multiplicity of types of goiter. The first of these types is known as colloid goiter, or endemic goiter, which is a development due directly to a lack of sufficient iodine levels. As a result, the people who tend to end up with a colloid goiter are those we mentioned, who live somewhere with a less dense supply of iodine.

The next type of goiter is the nontoxic goiter, or sporadic goiter, as it is also well known. Though the definite cause of a goiter of this type is regarded as generally unknown, it is surmised that a sporadic goiter is a result of taking medications, such as lithium, for example, or so it is believed. Among the may uses for lithium, it is perhaps most commonly recognized as the drug used for aiding in the treatment of mood based disorders, the likes of bipolar or depression. The nontoxic name is apt in regard to this form of goiter, as they are benign, and have no discernable effect on the production or secretion function of the thyroid gland, leaving the thyroid to function at a healthy and normal capacity.

The final type of commonly recognized goiter is known as the toxic nodular or multinodular goiter. Generally originating and taking form from as merely an extension from what was a simple goiter prior, the toxic nodular goiter will take the form of at least one, but often more, small nodules on the expanding thyroid gland. This toxic nodular goiter, having taken a sort of root on the thyroid gland, then begins to produce its own thyroid hormone, which plays a big part in the causation of hyperthyroidism.

As mentioned above, it can be difficult to detect goiter before it has really taken effect to the thyroid gland, but after it has begun doing it's work it is most common for it to cause a swelling of the front of the neck, making it clearly visible as well as felt. Before the expanding has commenced, it is common to have had nodules existing in your thyroid gland, these small nodules cannot be felt, and may have even been only a chance occurrence due to examinations, and of scans, that were applied for other reasons. Cases such as these are rather common, and when they occur, there has been a tendency to notice no sign of a goiter up to that point. As nodules appear on the thyroid, ranging from smaller nodules to much larger nodules, it is the presence of these nodules which is what is the cause of noticeable swelling of the neck.

This swelling and the nodules which are collecting on the thyroid gland cause other symptoms to occur, like having a difficult time of swallowing or of trying to breathe, it is not uncommon for coughing to be a symptom, your voice may start to become hoarse, and there may be a dizzy sensation that is noticeable when you raise an arm above your head.

Goiter is a rather common occurrence. It is calculated by the World Health Organization, that around the world, goiter affects nearly 12 percent of the global population. However, it has also been recorded that in Europe, the rate of goiter is lower by a slight amount. Goiter being considered endemic, or noticeably affecting a certain area is a common occurrence wherever iodine is scarce, and the endemic definitions are only applied when goiter is recognized on 1 out of 10 people within a certain population.

It is usual for goiter to be the diagnosis when there is noticeable swelling on the neck that can be seen without the need of a scan, also making it detectable with the touch of the hand, due to the enlarged thyroid gland in your neck, something a doctor will be quick to check for, likely before anything else.

There are also a number tests a general practitioner may order in order to examine the levels in your blood of thyroid hormones coming from the thyroid gland, as well as wanting to make sure of the levels of antibodies that are prevalent in the bloodstream. This examination will often take the form of blood tests, that are used to detect the changes in levels of the hormones as well as whether or not the level of production of the antibodies has increased, which tends to happen in response to the body experiencing an injury or infection in the blood.

A thyroid scan, or thyroid uptake scan, will show the size of the goiter itself, as well as what condition the goiter is in. It will also aid in identifying any differences in activity, in various places on the thyroid gland.

A biopsy may be recommended, the procedure of which involves removing samples of your thyroid gland, and then sending the samples of your thyroid gland's tissue to an outside laboratory or endocrinologist for examination.

It is also possible that an ultrasound scan may be used which will help for a doctor to see images of the inside of your neck, getting a much closer look at the size of the invasive goiter, allowing for the observation of nodules. As more ultrasounds are done, it is even then possible to track the changes in size or shape of the nodules, and the size of the goiter.

You may, at some point, be referred to an endocrinologist in order to get an outpatient assessment, giving you and the doctor more information from the examination by an expert. During their examination you may have to undergo a test known as a fine needle aspiration, which is done on the thyroid gland. For the procedure to take place, the endocrinologist will make use of a fine needle which, utilizing the guiding sight of an ultrasound, will be used to remove tissue from your thyroid gland, only a small amount will be needed. The tissue removed from your thyroid gland is then studied under the lens of a microscope, which will assist the endocrinologist in assessing exactly the types of cells which are currently present in your thyroid gland. It is not at all uncommon for a procedure like this to need to be repeated one or more times, for the sake of reaching an accurate result and helping you on your way to treatment and recovery.

There is no one, cut and dry, blanket method for treating a goiter, as the treatment will depend entirely on precisely what is the cause that is underlying the goiter. As well, a particular course of action will be decided by your doctor on the basis of the size of the goiter, and the condition that the goiter is in, as well as the symptoms you have that are associated with the goiter. It will also be important to not overlook any factors to your health that may have been responsible for the goiters formation when looking into treatment options.

A goiter which can be regarded as simple, having a prevalence of causing no imbalances in the thyroid gland, as well as no seeming problems as a result of the thyroid gland, will be less likely to cause further obstructions or overall issues.

In order to shrink a goiter, in the case of hypo or hyperthyroidism, it may be enough to just take prescribed medicines as a treatment for the symptoms and for the swelling of the thyroid gland. Medications which are known as corticosteroids often see use in the task of reducing any inflammation, or when there is a prevalence of thyroiditis.

Medicinal treatments for a goiter are not always the most effective response, however. It is not at all uncommon for a goiter to have grown too large to be able to respond properly to medicinal therapy and begin to shrink. In such a case there are surgeries which are available, known as a thyroidectomy. Undergoing a thyroidectomy will mean removing your thyroid gland completely and is a common option for when the thyroid gland grows too large and further obstructs what would otherwise be simple actions, such as swallowing or breathing.

When you are going through the experience of trying to treat what is the most harmful of the goiter family, the toxic nodular or multinodular goiter, RAI, or radioactive iodine treatment is typically the necessary response. You will be given a tablet, the RAI, which is a small amount of the radioactive iodine, which gets ingested orally and begins the process of destroying thyroid gland tissue.

When it comes to the treatment of a goiter, there are options for home care which can be very helpful and ought not to be overlooked as such. When you have finished up with all the treatment that can be offered at the hospital, or by a referred endocrinologist, it is an entirely common possibility that a discussion with your general practitioner will end in him or her suggesting you continue care of yourself in the home, with a prescription of some form of medication, which may end up being a decrease or increase in the amounts of iodine that you are ingesting regularly. This will, of course, be determined by the type of goiter that was ailing you, as well as requiring regular testing to keep an eye on your iodine levels, and the efficiency of your thyroid glands production and secretion of hormones. If it all ends up that a goiter is non-problematic, being too small to count as an issue or cause an imbalance, you may require no treatment or care at home at all.

100 Recipes for Acid Reflux

Although the names of some of the recipes in this chapter may be familiar, the **ingredients** used and style of preparation are what make them conducive to people who have issues with acid reflux.

1. Baked Chicken Parmesan

Total servings: 4

The **ingredients** to Use

- 4 chicken breasts with the bones and skin removed
- 4 tsp of olive oil
- ½ cup of breadcrumbs, seasoned
- 3 tbsp of Parmesan cheese, grated
- Salt to taste
- Italian seasoning to taste

How to Prepare The Meal

1. Make sure your oven is preheated to 375°F.
2. Grease a baking dish with vegetable cooking spray.
3. Place the Parmesan cheese and bread crumbs into a small bowl. Also, add salt and seasoning to taste, and mix the contents of the bowl well.
4. Place your chicken breasts on a cutting board and, using paper towels, pat them dry. Now coat the

chicken breasts with the olive oil before dredging each chicken in the Parmesan cheese mixture. Make sure to get every side of the chicken covered.

5. Place the chicken breasts on the greased baking dish. If there is anything left of the grated cheese and breadcrumb mixture, sprinkle it over the chicken breasts.

6. Place the baking dish in the oven uncovered, and let the chicken bake for about 40 minutes or until done. Use a meat thermometer to test. Chicken should be at least 165°F.

2. Chicken Pot Pie

Total servings: 4

The **Ingredients** to Use

- 1 pound of chicken breasts with the bones and skin removed

- 1 cup of biscuit mix

- 1 tbsp olive oil

- ¾ cup of skimmed milk

- 1 can of creamed corn

- 1 cup of carrots that have been frozen, thawed, and drained

- 1 cup of peas that have been frozen, thawed, and drained

- ½ tsp of salt

How to Prepare The Meal

1. Preheat your oven to 400°F.

2. Dice the chicken breasts into little cubes and add ½ tsp of salt to season it.

3. Place your skillet over medium-high heat and add olive oil. Heat the oil in the pan for about 8 seconds before adding the chicken breasts. Cook for about 9 minutes or until the cubes are brown.

4. Place your chicken into a baking dish and add your carrots. Cover the baking dish, put it in your preheated oven, and bake for 25 minutes.

5. In a medium to large mixing bowl add the skimmed milk and biscuit mix into it. Mix them together until they form a dough.

6. Once your chicken breast cubes are well baked, take out the baking dish and spread the dough onto both chicken and carrots.

7. Put the baking dish back in the oven and bake for an additional 10 minutes.

3. Chicken Noodle Soup

Total servings: 4

The **Ingredients** to Use

- 2 cups of frozen peas

- ½ tbsp of olive oil

- 2 cups of cooked and chopped chicken breasts with the bones and skin removed

- 1 cup of diced celery

- 3 ounces of uncooked egg noodles

- 2 quarts of water

- 4 chicken bouillon cubes, low-sodium

- 2 cups of carrots, peeled and diced

- ½ tsp of thyme

- ½ tsp of salt

How to Prepare The Meal

1. Into a large pot, add the olive oil and celery. Set your stove to medium-high heat and sauté the celery.

2. When the celery is translucent, put your water, carrots, chicken cubes, thyme and salt in the pot. Let the mixture boil for about 9 minutes, until the noodles have softened.

3. Next, add chicken breasts and frozen peas. Reduce the heat to medium-low and let the contents of the pot boil for 10 minutes.

4. Quinoa Stuffed Chicken Roll-ups

Total servings: 4

The **Ingredients** to Use

- ½ lemon, the zest
- 2 tbsp dry quinoa
- 2 tbsp crumbled feta cheese
- Medium carrot, halved and julienned
- ¼ cup of julienned broccoli stalks
- ½ cup of chopped spinach
- 2 medium pounded chicken breasts with the bones and skin removed
- ¼ tsp of salt
- ¼ tsp of dry oregano

How to Prepare The Meal

1. Cook your quinoa according to the **directions** on the package.
2. Make sure your oven is preheated to 350°F. Next, steam your broccoli and carrots. Stop when they are tender.
3. Line a baking sheet with paper towels and place the chicken breasts on it. Coat the chicken in olive oil and rub salt on all sides.

4. Divide carrots, spinach, broccoli, quinoa, and oregano between both of the chicken. Then add lemon zest and feta cheese. With a spoon, gather everything to the middle of the pounded chicken and begin rolling it. Roll to the end and close the chicken with a toothpick.

5. Set your stove to medium-low heat. Cook the roll-ups for about 5 minutes, by which time they must have turned brown.

6. Put the chicken rolls back on the baking sheet. Bake for 15 minutes before taking it out.

7. Remember to allow some time for the chicken to slightly cool before cutting it.

5. Chicken and Red Potatoes

Total servings: 4

The **Ingredients** to Use

- 2 large carrots, chopped
- 2 limes, thinly chopped
- 1 tbsp of melted butter
- 2 tbsp of fresh parsley
- 300 grams of red potatoes that have been diced into little cubes
- 2 tbsp of apple cider vinegar
- ½ tsp of dried rosemary
- 2 cups of grilled chicken, shredded
- ⅓ cups of green olives, pitted
- ¼ tsp of turmeric
- ¼ tsp of salt

How to Prepare The Meal

1. Make sure your oven is heated to 425°F.

2. In a large bowl, put your turmeric, potatoes, carrots, salt, and melted butter. Toss these well before spreading them on a rimmed baking sheet. Also, squeeze the juice from your limes onto the baking sheet. Leave the baking sheet uncovered and put it

in the oven. Bake for 35 minutes, by which time the carrots and potatoes should have softened.

3. Get your casserole dish and put your baked cooked carrots and potatoes in it. Also add apple cider vinegar, rosemary, shredded chicken, and olives. Stir the contents of the casserole dish together.

4. Let them cook for 15 minutes.

6. Strawberry and Balsamic Vinegar Semifreddo

Total servings: 4

The **Ingredients** to Use

- 4 small strawberries
- Water (about 85 ml)
- 1 tsp of Manuka honey
- 2 tbsp of Balsamic vinegar
- 150 grams of ripe strawberries
- 4 fresh mint sprigs

How to Prepare The Meal

1. Preset your freezer to rapid freeze. You should do this at least 2 hours before you put your finished dinner in the freezer.

2. In a saucepan, add the honey and water. Set your stove to medium and boil the honey and water mixture. Stir occasionally. Reduce the heat to low before adding strawberries. Let it boil for another 4 minutes before taking your pan from the heat.

3. Turn the contents of your pan into a food processor. Also add the balsamic vinegar. Process this for 30 to 35 seconds.

4. In a freeze-proof dish pour the mixture in the food processor into it. Put this in you preset freezer and let it cool for about 1 hour and 25 minutes. Stir twice during this process.

5. You'll need 4 dessert glasses, and use a scoop to take the semi-frozen mixture (semifreddo) and put it in each glass. Slice your strawberries in half and put 2 halves into each glass. Also, add mint sprigs.

As a side note, your freezer was set to rapid freeze for the semifreddo. Return it to its normal setting once you are done.

7. Poached Eggs with Spinach

Total servings: 2

The **Ingredients** to Use

- 2 toasted slices of whole grain bread

- 4 cold jumbo eggs

- 1 bunch spinach

- 3 tsp of apple cider vinegar

- Kosher salt to taste

- Water

How to Prepare The Meal

1. Pour water in a skillet, up to 1 inch of the pan. Then add a pinch of salt and apple cider vinegar. Set the pan over medium heat and let it boil.

2. Break your eggs into 4 custard dishes and pour each of them into the water in the skillet. Next, turn the stove off and cover the skillet. Set it aside for 5 minutes.

3. Using a slotted spoon, remove the eggs from the skillet after the allotted 5 minutes.

4. Place the poached eggs on your neatly arranged "bed" of spinach. It is ready to be served with your toasted slices of bread.

8. Cottage Cheese Salsa with Starfruit Slices

Total servings: 6

The **Ingredients** to Use

- 2 tbsp of basil, chopped into ribbon-like shapes

- 16 oz of low-fat cottage cheese

- 1 sliced large starfruit

- 150 grams of papaya, deseeded and chopped

How to Prepare The Meal

1. In a bowl, place your papaya, cottage cheese, and basil. Mix them well together.

2. Place each slice of starfruit on a flat plate. With a scoop, put some of the cottage cheese mixture on the starfruit slices. To prevent the mixture from sliding off the starfruits, you may want to dry each slice of starfruit first.

9. Watermelon and Cantaloupe Parfait

Total servings: 4

The **Ingredients** to Use

- 1 cup of watermelon, deseeded and chopped

- 1 cup of sweet cantaloupe, diced

- 1 small peeled apple, with the core removed and diced

- 16 oz of unsweetened low-fat yogurt, whipped

- 2 cups of low-fat granola

How to Prepare The Meal

1. Separate your cantaloupe equally among 4 clean parfait glasses. Then, top each glass with ¼ cups of yogurt and granola. Yogurt before the granola.

2. Place equal amounts of your chopped apples in each glass. Like before, top each parfait glasses with the same measurement (¼ cups) of yogurt and granola.

3. Separate your diced watermelon among the 4 glasses.

4. Finally, top with a generous amount of yogurt and granola.

10. Polenta with Sesame Seeds

Total servings: 1

The **Ingredients** to Use

- 1 tbsp of sesame seeds

- ¾ cup of instant polenta

- 2 cups of water

- Salt to desired taste

- ½ tsp of vanilla extract

- 1 cup of almond milk

- 1 tsp Manuka honey

- 1 tsp of orange extract

How to Prepare The Meal

1. Place the milk into a medium pot and boil over medium heat.

2. Add polenta into the milk and whisk thoroughly.

3. Let it boil until the mixture is thick and creamy before adding sugar, orange extract, vanilla, salt.

4. Put into a bowl, sprinkle sesame seeds on it, and your meal is ready to be served.

11. Turkey and Plum Bites

Total servings: 4

The **Ingredients** to Use

- 115 grams of shredded pak choi

- 140 grams of chopped turkey steaks with the skin removed

- 4 small onions

- 1 small deseeded yellow pepper, thinly chopped into strips

- 2 stoned ripe plums, diced into 4 even with

- 1 that of olive oil

- 2 tbsp of plum sauce

- 2 than of orange juice

How to Prepare The Meal

1. Line your grill with thin foil and make sure it is preheated to high.

2. With 4 skewers, thread the turkeys. Do this alongside the onions and plums.

3. In a small bowl, place the plum sauce and orange juice. Mix these together and coat your turkey kebabs. Set it aside to marinate for 15-20 minutes.

4. Cook the turkey on the grill for 10 minutes. Turn it halfway into the 10 minutes to ensure both sides are cooked.

5. Heat a wok, adding some oil to the pan. Put in your yellow pepper and stir for 2 minutes. Add what is left of your orange juice and plum sauce, and continue stirring. Finally, add the pak choi and let it cook for 1 minute.

12. Turkey Burgers

Total servings: 8

The **Ingredients** to Use

- 1 tbsp of butter

- 55 grams of long grain white rice

- ½ tsp of allspice, ground

- 450 grams of lean turkey, minced

- ½ tsp of dried thyme

- 1 small apple, which has been cored, peeled, and grated

- 1 tsp of sage

- 1 tsp of onion powder

- all1 tsp of garlic powder

How to Prepare The Meal

1. In a large pot, put some water into it to boil. Add white rice to boiling water and let it cook for about 10 minutes. At this time, your rice should be soft enough to be edible, but not mushy.

2. Drain the rice with a colander. You can add some cold water to the rice and drain it again to remove excess starch.

3. In a large bowl add the rice, ground allspice, minced turkey, dried thyme, grated apple, sage, onion powder, and garlic powder inside it. Mix them.

4. Wash your hands and mold this mixture into the shape of 8 burger patties.

5. Place a non-stick skillet over medium-high heat and put your butttin it. Cook your patties in it for 10 minutes, turning it halfway through to get all the sides.

13. Gingered Prawn Wraps

Total servings: 4

The **Ingredients** to Use

- 140 grams of peeled carrots
- 225 grams of peeled and deveined prawns
- 3 trimmed celery sticks
- 2 tsp of grated lime rind
- ½ peeled cucumber
- 1 deseeded red pepper
- 2 tbsp of lime juice
- 8 large lettuce leaves
- 1 inch ginger, grated
- 1 tbsp of olive oil
- 1 tsp of garlic powder
- Ground pepper to desired taste

How to Prepare The Meal

1. Cut the carrot, red pepper, celery, and cucumber into thin strips. Put these in a large plate, alongside your lettuce leaves (separately), and set them aside.

2. Set a skillet over medium heat and put your olive oil in it. Add your prawns and ginger, and let it cook for 1 minute. Next, add your garlic powder, grated lime

rind, and lime juice into the pan. Continue to cook and stir occasionally for 4 minutes. By that time, your prawns should have achieved a pinkish color. Add some pepper.

3. Put some of those vegetables onto each lettuce leaf and place a prawn on each one.

14. Crisp Bread Bruschetta

Total servings: 4

The **Ingredients** to Use

- ¼ of a small apple, thinly chopped

- ½ of a small melon, diced into wedges

- 8 crispbreads

- 8 cucumber slices

- 4 tsp of low-fat cream cheese, preferably the herb flavored kind

- 8 raspberries

- 55 grams of rocket leaves

- 150 grams of lean boiled ham, sliced

- 4 cherry tomatoes, each cut in half

- Pepper to preferred taste

How to Prepare The Meal

1. On the crispbreads, spread the cream cheese and add rocket leaves on each bread. Also, arrange your melons on the bread before topping with the slices of ham.

2. Place your raspberry, cucumber, and apple on top. Sprinkle pepper to desired taste, and your appetizer is ready to be served.

15. Prawn and Mango Salad

Total servings: 4

The **Ingredients** to Use

For the salad, you need:

- Mixes leaves (kale, lettuce, cabbage, and any other preferred salad leaf)

- 250 grams of peeled and deveined prawns, cooked

- 2 large mangoes

For the dressing, you need:

- 1 tbsp of lemon juice

- Mango juice

- 6 tbsp of low-fat yogurt

- Salt and pepper to desired taste

How to Prepare The Meal

1. Slice the mango on both sides. Don't cut too close to the seed. With each slice, cut little cubes and remove the skin. Make sure to catch the mango juices in a bowl. Put the mango cubes in a larger bowl and add prawns.

2. Put yogurt, lemon juice, salt, and pepper inside the bowl of mango juice and mix well.

3. On a serving dish, place your salad leaves. Add the mango and prawn on top of it and drizzle with the contents of the smaller bowl.

16. Chicken Sesame Kebab

Total servings: 4

The **Ingredients** to Use

- 3 tbsp of low-fat yogurt

- 200 grams of chicken breasts with the bones removed and flesh cut into thin strips

- 1 tbsp of sesame seeds

- 3 tbsp of lemon juice

- 6 small radishes, sliced

- 1 large grated carrot

- 1 tbsp of low-sodium soy sauce

- 1 thinly sliced red onions

- 1 tsp of Manuka honey

- 175 grams of assorted salad leaves

How to Prepare The Meal

1. Preheat your grill. Set it to high.

2. Make sure your skewers are presoaked. Now, thread your boneless chicken breasts through the skewers.

3. In a small bowl, put your soy sauce, honey, and 2 tbsp of lemon juice. Mix them well together. Coat the chicken with this mixture and set it aside for 15 to 20 minutes to marinate.

4. On a large flat plate, arrange your salad leaves. Place your red onion slices and grate carrots on it.

5. Grill your skewered chicken breasts for 10 minutes and when you are done, sprinkle lots of sesame seeds on it.

6. In a small bowl, mix your yogurt and lemon juice and pour the mixture onto the salad.

17. Broiled Chicken Kebabs

Total servings: 4

The **Ingredients** to Use

- 1 cup of long-grain brown rice
- 1 ½ pounds of chicken breasts with the bones and skin removed
- 1 tbsp of olive oil
- 3 cups of small whole button mushrooms with the stems removed
- 1 tsp of oregano
- 4 cups of zucchini, chopped
- 1 tsp of basil
- 1 vegetable cooking spray
- ½ tsp rosemary
- ½ tsp parsley

How to Prepare The Meal

1. In a large bowl, cook the rice according to the **directions** on the pack.
2. In a medium bowl add the olive oil, parsley, basil, rosemary, and oregano.
3. Cut your chicken breasts into 1 inch pieces and put them in the bowl. Make sure all the sides are coated

in the mixture. Set it aside to marinate for 15 - 20 minutes. Wash the vegetables during this time.

4. Also, add your mushrooms and zucchini to the bowl and mix.

5. On all 8 skewers, thread chicken, mushrooms, and zucchinis.

6. Spray your broiler pan with your non-stick vegetable oil and place your chicken kebabs on it. Broil the kebabs for 5 minutes on each side.

7. Serve the chicken kebabs with the brown rice.

18. Balsamic Chicken Salad

Total serving: 4

The **Ingredients** to Use

- ½ cup of chopped parsley
- 2 cups of mixed salad leaves, chopped
- 4 diced chicken breasts, with the bones and skin removed
- A 15 oz can of lentils, rinsed
- 1 tbsp of butter
- 2 tbsp of apple juice
- ½ tsp of ginger powder
- 1 chopped green apple
- 2 thinly diced stalks of celery
- 2 tbsp of balsamic vinegar
- Salt and pepper to desired taste

How to Prepare The Meal

1. Place the diced chicken breasts in a bowl and season them with ginger and pepper.

2. Place a large skillet over medium heat and melt your butter. Next, put your chicken in the pan and cook for about 9 minutes. By this time, the chicken breasts should have turned a brown color.

3. After the 10 minutes, turn off the heat, remove the chicken from the pan and coat it with vinegar.

4. Toss celery, apple juice, celery, chopped green apples, and salt in a large bowl.

5. Also, add your lentils, salad leaves, parsley, and chicken breasts into the bowl and gently fold.

19. Blueberry and Cinnamon Oatmeal

Total servings: 1

The **Ingredients** to Use

- 1 tsp of chopped walnuts

- 1 cup of almond milk

- 1 tsp of Manuka honey

- ¼ cup of blueberries

- ⅔ cups of quick oats

- A full cup of water

- 1 tbsp of crushed flax seeds

- 1 tsp of vanilla extract

- 1 tsp of cinnamon, ground

How to Prepare The Meal

1. Heat some water in a pan before adding your oats.

2. Add flax seeds, vanilla extract, and cinnamon to the pan and stir. Keep stirring the oats until the water is no longer visible, and the oats are soft. This should take between 3 to 5 minutes.

3. Next, add almond milk and blueberries, and stir.

4. Pour your oatmeal into a bowl. Mix in honey and top with walnuts.

20. Banana and Ginger Smoothie

Total servings: 2

The **Ingredients** to Use

- ½ cup of ice

- 2 cups of low-fat milk

- 2 small, ripe bananas

- 1 tbsp of honey

- 1 cup of unsweetened yogurt

- ½ tsp of grated ginger

How to Prepare The Meal

1. Peel the skin from your banana and dice it into a blender. Then add the ginger, yogurt, ice, and milk. Blend until the mixture reaches a smooth consistency.

2. Add honey and blend for 10 seconds more.

21. Cheese and Egg Souffle

Total servings: 3

The **Ingredients** to Use

- 3 tbsp of shredded mozzarella cheese

- 3 jumbo eggs

- 2 tbsp of milk

- Freshly ground pepper

- Non-stick cooking spray

- Garlic salt to taste (preferably, a pinch)

How to Prepare The Meal

1. Preset your oven to 375°F

2. Place the milk, eggs, pepper, and salt in a bowl. Mix them well.

3. Get 3 ramekins and spray them with your cooking spray. Then add cheese into each ramekin, up to ½ of the glass bowls.

4. Fill the ramekins with the egg mixture in your bowl.

5. Place each of the glass bowls on a cookie sheet and bake the cheese for 30 minutes.

22. Mexican Egg Scramble

Total servings: 2

The **Ingredients** to Use

- 4 eggs jumbo

- 3 slices of bacon

- ½ cup of Mexican blend cheese

- 1 cup of chopped mushrooms

- ½ cup of chopped red peppers

- Salt and pepper

How to Prepare The Meal

1. Place a non-stick skillet over medium heat and cook your bacon to crispiness. Then take the bacon out and cut it in ½ inch pieces.

2. With the same oil, sauté your mushrooms and pepper for 5 minutes.

3. Break the eggs into the same pan and fry. Stir while doing so. Cook until they are done.

4. Next, stir in the cheese.

5. Put your bacon back in the pan and turn off the heat. Fold with the eggs.

23. Stewed Creamy Apple

Total servings: 4

The **Ingredients** to Use

- Few sprigs of mint

- 450 grams of diced cooking apples

- 140 grams of raspberries

- 1 tbsp of honey

- 300 ml of yogurt

- 1 tsp of ground cinnamon

- 3 tbsp of water

How to Prepare The Meal

1. In a saucepan, add cinnamon, honey, apples and water. Set your stove to low heat and cook for 15 minutes. Stir occasionally. Then, take your pan from the heat and beat the contents of the pan until you can no longer see lumps.

2. Place the yogurt in a large bowl and stir vigorously until it achieves a smooth consistency. Also, stir the cinnamon mixture and some of your raspberries into the yogurt.

3. With a spoon, put your yogurt mixture into four dishes and leave to cool down.

4. Decorate with mint sprigs and what's left of the raspberries.

24. Ruby Fruits with Meringue

Total servings: 4

The **Ingredients** to Use

For the meringue, you need:

- 40 grams of castor sugar

- 1 egg white

For the Ruby fruit, you need:

- Some fresh mint sprigs

- 225 grams of strawberries

- 350 grams of mixed fruit, which could include cherries with stones, blackcurrants, strawberries, and raspberries

- 2 tsp of clear honey

- 200 ml of water

How to Prepare The Meal

1. Ensure that your oven is preheated to 250°F.

2. Get a medium-sized bowl (grease free) and put egg whites in it. Whisk it to stiffness, all the while adding a spoonful of sugar (all 40 grams).

3. When this is done, spoon the mixture into a piping bag and make little swirl shapes with it on a lined baking sheet.

4. Put it in your oven for about 1 hour, by which time the mounds should have become crisp.

5. Turn off the oven and leave it to cool down.

6. Place the honey, water, and strawberries in a saucepan over medium-low heat, and boil for 8 minutes. Turn off the stove and set the saucepan aside for 5 minutes.

7. Put the strawberries in a food processor and make it into a puree.

8. Pass the puree through a sieve and prepare the mixed fruits.

9. Stir the puree into the fruits. Serve topped with meringue.

25. Fruity Stuffed Nectarines

Total servings: 4

The **Ingredients** to Use

- 1 tbsp of grated orange rind

- 1 tsp of Manuka oil

- 4 nectarines

- 200 ml of low-fat yogurt

- 140 grams of blueberries

- 150 ml of freshly made orange juice

- 115 grams of raspberries

How to Prepare The Meal

1. Make sure your oven is preheated to 350°F.

2. Cut each nectarine in half and remove their stones. Then, place them in an oven-proof dish.

3. Put some blueberries and raspberries into a bowl. Break and mix them together. Fill the holes of each nectarine with the mixture.

4. Also, mix orange juice and honey in a bowl. Drip it over the nectarine.

5. Blend your grated orange rind and yogurt. After this, pour the content of your blender into a bowl and keep it in a refrigerator.

6. Put the nectarines in your oven and bake for 10 minutes.

7. Your dessert is ready to be served. You may eat it with some of the cold grated orange rind and yogurt mixture spooned over the nectarines.

26. Aromatic Pears

Total servings: 4

The **Ingredients** to Use

- 300 ml of water

- 4 ripe pears

- 2 fresh bay leaves

- 2 tbsp of lemon juice

- 2 whole cloves

- 1 tbsp of honey

- 1 average sized (1 cm) root ginger, peeled and dice

- 2 whole star anise

- 1 bruised stalk of lemongrass

- 1 bruised cinnamon stick

How to Prepare The Meal

1. Peel the skin off your pears without damaging their stalk. Next, put them in a bowl and pour lemon juice over them.

2. In a large saucepan add honey, water, cinnamon stick, bay leaf, ginger, cloves, star anise, and lemon grass. Place the pan over medium-low heat and stir occasionally. When you can no longer see the honey, drain your pears and add them to the

contents of the pan. Reduce the heat to low and continue boiling for another 20 minutes.

3. Turn off the heat and take the pears from the pan. Continue boiling the syrup in the pan for another 8 minutes. When it has thickened, set it aside to cool down for about 10 minutes before pouring it over the pears.

27. Mixed Bean Soup

Total servings: 4

The **Ingredients** to Use

- 400 grams of pre-soaked red kidney beans

- 1 tsp of garlic powder

- 400 grams of pre-soaked black-eyed beans

- 1 tsp of grass-fed butter

- 1 tbsp of mixed dried herbs

- 1 large chopped tomatoes

- 600 ml of vegetable stock

- 2 bay leaves

- 1 diced carrot

- 1 diced celery stalk

- Crusty bread, if you prefer

- 1 tbsp of balsamic vinegar

How to Prepare The Meal

1. Drain your kidney and black-eyed beans and rinse them. Place them in a stock pot and add your vegetable stock and bay leaves. Cook for 1 hour and 30 minutes.

2. Next, add chopped celery stalk, tomatoes, carrots, and balsamic vinegar into the pot. Reduce the heat

to low and cook for another 20 minutes. You may add water to the beans so make it as thick or watery as your like.

3. Mix in garlic, dried herbs, and butter and cook for 5 more minutes.

4. You may serve with crusty bread.

28. Tilapia with Cucumber Salsa and Brown Rice

Total servings: 4

The **Ingredients** to Use

- 1 cup of long-grain brown rice
- 4 tilapia filets
- 1 chopped small English cucumber
- 2 tbsp of pineapple juice
- 1 chopped spring onion
- 1 tbsp of grated ginger
- ¼ cup of chopped pineapple
- 1 tbsp of honey
- 1 tbsp of coconut oil
- ¼ tsp of pepper
- 2 tbsp of olive oil

How to Prepare The Meal

1. Cook the rice according to the **directions** on the pack.

2. In a large bowl place the ginger, pineapple juice, olive oil, honey, spring onions, pepper, pineapple chunks, and chopped cucumber.

3. Place a skillet over medium heat and put coconut oil in it. Sprinkle your tilapia with pepper and sauté both sides for 3 minutes each.

4. Serve your tilapia with the brown rice.

29. Pan seared tilapia

Total servings: 4

The **Ingredients** to Use

- 6 oz tilapia filets (4 of them)

- 1 cup of long-grain rice

- 2 ½ tbsp of olive oil

- 2 tbsp pineapple juice

- ¼ cup of chopped red pepper

- 2 tsp of honey

- 1 tbsp of grated ginger

- 1 chopped small English cucumber

- 1 pound canned pineapple pieces

- Salt and pepper to desired taste

How to Prepare The Meal

1. Cook your rice in accordance with the **directions** on the pack.

2. In a medium-sized bowl, mix pineapple juice, honey, ginger, and 2 tbsp of olive oil. Next, add the chopped cucumber, pineapple, and pepper.

3. Get a large non-stick and heat 1 tsp of olive oil in it.

4. Sprinkle and season your tilapia filets with ¼ salt and pepper.

5. Cook it on your skillet for 3 minutes. Ensure you cook both sides of the tilapia.

6. Serve with your rice and pineapple mixture.

30. Asparagus and Green Bean Salad

Total servings: 12

The **Ingredients** to Use

- 3 tbsp of olive oil

- 1 pound of asparagus

- 4 tsp of balsamic vinegar

- 1 pound of French beans with the stem removed

- 1 tsp of Dijon mustard

- 2 tbsp of carrots, shredded

- 4 slices of cooked turkey bacon, crumbled

- 3 hard-boiled eggs, quartered

- Salt and pepper to taste

How to Prepare The Meal

1. Place a large pot containing water over medium-low heat and boil your beans and asparagus for 4 minutes.

2. Next, drain the beans and asparagus, and rinse them. Place them in a container and set aside in your fridge.

3. Place the Dijon mustard, balsamic vinegar, olive oil, salt, and pepper in a bowl and whisk. This is your vinaigrette.

4. Remove the beans and asparagus from the fridge and put them in a salad bowl. Sprinkle your carrots and crumbled bacon over them.

5. Pour your vinaigrette over it and place your quartered eggs on top.

31. Black Bean Burger

Total servings: 6

The **Ingredients** to Use

- 6 buns, whole wheat

- 2 drained 15 oz cans of black beans

- 1 iceberg lettuce

- ⅓ cup of green peppers, chopped

- 2 tbsp of flour

- Some pineapple slices, divided

- 2 tbsp of minced cilantro

- ¼ cup of vegetable oil

- 1 tsp of cumin, ground

- ½ cup of baked and crushed tortilla chips

- ½ tsp of coriander, ground

- Salt and pepper

How to Prepare The Meal

1. Get a baking sheet and line it with paper towels and place 1 can of your drained beans on it. Spread them out. Set it aside for 20 minutes.

2. Add the second can of drained beans to a bowl containing eggs, flour, the various seasonings, and tortilla chips.

3. Mold them into patties and keep them in your refrigerator.

4. Get a non-stick skillet and heat your vegetable oil in it. Cook 3 burgers in the pan for 5 minutes. Flip the burgers to ensure you cook both sides.

5. Remove them and set aside.

6. Serve them on your buns and place pineapple slices as toppings.

32. Banana Walnut Muffins

Total servings: 18

The **Ingredients** to Use

- ½ cup of dried unsweetened coconut, grated
- 2 cups of whole wheat flour
- ½ cup of walnuts, chopped
- 1 tsp of salt
- 1 tsp of vanilla extract
- 1 ½ tsp of baking powder
- 3 ripe bananas, mashed
- ¾ cups of sugar
- 2 eggs
- ⅓ cup of coconut oil

How to Prepare The Meal

1. Ensure that your oven is preheated to 375°F. Grease a muffin tin.

2. Place the grated coconut, wheat flour, salt, and baking powder in a bowl. Mix them.

3. Then, mix oil, eggs, and your mashed bananas in another bowl.

4. Pour the egg mixture into the bowl of flour and baking powder, and mix then well.

5. Add grated coconut, vanilla, and walnuts to the bowl and stir.

6. Place them in muffin tins, almost filling them (⅔)

7. Bake for 18 minutes. To know if the muffin is cooked, put a toothpick in it. Should it come out clean, then the muffin is ready. Set them aside to cool for 5 minutes.

33. Crockpot Chicken and Barley Stew

Total servings: 6

The **Ingredients** to Use

- 2 cups of small chopped spinach

- 2 chicken breasts

- 2 bay leaves

- ¾ cup or barley

- 2 tsp of oregano, basil, and thyme

- 48 oz of chicken broth, low in sodium

- 1 small onion, chopped

- A 16 oz bag of frozen vegetables, mixed

- ¼ tsp of garlic powder

- Salt and pepper to preferred taste

How to Prepare The Meal

1. Place all the **ingredients** in a crockpot, but set your spinach aside.

2. Mix to ensure everything is beneath your chicken broth.

3. Reduce the heat of the crockpot to low, cover it, and cook. It will take about 6 hours for the barley to be tender.

4. 30 minutes before the 6 hours is complete, add the spinach.

5. After the 6 hours, take out the bay leaves.

6. Also, take the chicken breasts from the soup, shred them before adding back to the pot.

7. Turn off the heat and your meal is ready.

34. Chicken Cutlets with Sautéed Mushrooms

Total servings: 4

The **Ingredients** to Use

- ⅓ cup of white wine

- 1 pound of chicken breast cutlets

- 2 cups of sliced mushrooms

- ⅓ cup of whole wheat flour

- 3 tbsp of butter

- 2 that of olive oil

- Salt and pepper to preferred taste

How to Prepare The Meal

1. Sprinkle and rub salt and pepper into the chicken cutlets.

2. Put your whole wheat flour into a large bowl and lightly coat your chicken.

3. In a large skillet placed over medium-high heat, heat your olive oil. Next, place your floured chicken cutlets into the pan and cook each side for 4 minutes or until both sides attain a golden brown color.

4. After this, take the chicken from the pan and set it aside. Reduce the heat of the stove to medium and

add mushrooms and butter to the pan. Sauté for 5 minutes.

5. Add your white wine to the pan and stir so it is deglazed.

6. Put the chicken cutlets back in the pan and continue cooking for 3 minutes.

35. Marinated Portobello Mushroom Sandwich

Total servings: 4

The **Ingredients** to Use

- ¼ cup of crumbled feta cheese

- 12 oz of Portobello mushrooms

- ⅓ cup of olive oil

- ¼ cup of basil, thinly diced

- ¼ cup of balsamic vinegar

- ¼ cup of sun-dried tomatoes, drained and diced

- 2 minced cloves of garlic

- 4 rolls of and sandwich you prefer. We'll use ciabatta in this recipe.

- 1 cup of yellow onions, diced

How to Prepare The Meal

1. Dampen a paper towel and clean the mushrooms. In a resealable plastic bag place your mushrooms, oil, garlic, vinegar, and onion. Set aside in the refrigerator to marinate for at least an hour. You can leave it for up to two days to properly marinate.

2. Ensure your oven is preheated to 375°F. Slice your ciabatta rolls and place them on a baking sheet.

3. Set your stove to medium-high and put all the contents of your plastic bag in the pan. Cook and stir for 15 minutes.

4. Put the rolls in the oven and bake for about 8 minutes. They should have a crispy feel to them.

5. Pour the mixture in your pan onto your rolls and place your tomatoes, feta cheese crumbles, and basil on top of the rolls.

36. Asparagus Quiche

Total servings: 8

The **Ingredients** to Use

- ⅛ tsp of nutmeg

- 1 9-inch pie crust, unbaked

- ¼ cup of Parmesan cheese

- ½ pound of chopped asparagus (¼ inch)

- ½ cup of Swiss cheese

- 6 cooked turkey bacon strips, diced

- 2 tbsp of green onions

- 1 ½ cup of low-fat yogurt

- 3 eggs

How to Prepare The Meal

1. Make sure your oven is preheated to 375°F.

2. Cover your unbaked pie crust with aluminum foil and let it bake for 5 minutes. Take off the foil and bake for another 5 minutes.

3. Steam your asparagus for about 5 minutes. It should have attained a bright green color without losing its crispness.

4. Break your eggs into a bowl and beat them. Add your yogurt slowly and carefully into the bowl. Also, add onions, nutmeg and salt.

5. Also, add most of your Parmesan and Swiss cheese. What is left will be used later.

6. Add your cooked bacon to the bowl of eggs and yogurt.

7. At the bottom of the pie crust, spread your steamed asparagus.

8. Drizzle your egg mixture over the asparagus and sprinkle your remaining Parmesan and Swiss cheese over it.

9. Reduce the heat of your oven to 350°F and bake for 40 minutes. To know that your quiche is finished, put a knife in the center. If it comes out clean, then the quiche is ready.

10. Set the quiche aside for about 15 minutes before serving.

37. Whole Wheat Banana Walnut Scones

Total servings: 8

The **Ingredients** to Use

- ¼ cup of chocolate chips (this is optional)

- 1 ¼ cup of oatmeal

- ¼ cup of walnut pieces

- 1 ¼ cup of whole wheat flour

- ¼ cup of brown sugar

- 1 banana, mashed

- 2 tbsp of flax seeds, ground

- ⅔ cup of plain yogurt, the non-fat kind

- 1 tsp of baking powder

- ½ cup of smart balance

- ½ tsp of baking soda

How to Prepare The Meal

1. Ensure your oven is preheated to 400°F.

2. Put the oatmeal, brown sugar, flour, flax seeds, baking powder, and baking soda into a bowl and mix. Using a pastry blender, cut the smart balance into the bowl.

3. Add yogurt and mashed bananas to the mixture, and stir. Also, throw in your walnuts and chocolate chips.

4. Scoop from the banana mixture to make 8 scones.

5. Line a cookie sheet with wax paper or parchment paper and place your scones on it.

6. Bake for 18 minutes.

38. Whole Wheat Empanadas

Total servings: 14

The **Ingredients** to Use

- 5 tbsp of water

- 3 cups of whole wheat flour (white)

- 1 egg

- 6 oz of unsalted butter, cut in 1 ½ lines

- ¼ tsp of salt

How to Prepare The Meal

1. Ensure your oven is preheated to 375°F.

2. Use a food processor to mix the salt and flour. Also, add your egg, butter, and water into the food processor and continue mixing until it forms a dough.

3. Take this dough and make a ball with it. Then, flatten it on wax or parchment paper and refrigerate for about 30 minutes.

4. Take the dough from the refrigerator, roll it into a ball and, using a mold, cut the round shapes to be used for the empanadas.

5. Put a tbsp of filling at the center of the dough (with respect to the size of the round shapes you cut) and fold them.

6. With your fingers, shape the edges into the decoration associated with empanadas.

7. To make the top golden, brush it with egg wash.

8. Bake your empanadas for 25 minutes or until done.

39. Pot Pie

Total servings: 8

The **Ingredients** to Use

For the crust, you need:

- 1 cup of Smart Balance butter (you can substitute the brand)
- 1 cup of whole wheat flour
- 6 tbsp of water
- 1 cup of all-purpose flour
- ½ tsp of salt

For the filling, we need:

- ⅓ cup of all-purpose flour
- 3 cups of shredded chicken
- 1 cup of chicken stock, low-sodium
- 2 cups of diced potatoes
- ⅔ cups of milk
- 1 cup of peas, asparagus, carrots, and corn with salt added to the mixture.
- ⅓ cup of Smart Balance butter
- ⅓ cup of green onions
- ⅓ cup of chopped celery

How to Prepare The Meal

1. Make sure your oven is preheated to 425°F.

2. To prepare the crust, mix salt and flour in a bowl. Cut in your butter and spread with a knife until it looks like coarse crumbs.

3. Sprinkle some water (1 ½ tsp) over the dough and fold it over the water. The dryness of the dough may necessitate the addition of more water.

4. Next, mold the dough into the shape of a ball and keep it in your refrigerator for 30 minutes.

5. Place your saucepan over medium heat and add some butter to it. Sauté your celery and green onions. Add salt, ⅓ of flour, and pepper. Also, add milk and broth. Stir occasionally to thicken the mixture.

6. Next, put in your meat, mixed vegetables, and potatoes. Now, turn your stove off.

7. Take your dough from the refrigerator and cut it in half.

8. Flatten each half of dough against 2 pieces of wax paper. Roll the dough until it is about ⅛ inch thick.

9. For one half of your dough, put it in your pie pan. Also, put your filling in the pan. With the top of the crust, cover both the bottom crust and filling.

10. To allow steam a chance to escape, make some cuts on top of the dough. The cuts should be little more than slits.

11. Bake in your preheated oven for 40 minutes. The crust should have turned brown. Also, the potatoes should be tender.

12. Take the pot pie out leave it for 5 minutes to set. This is to ensure it doesn't fall apart.

40. Stuffed Mushroom Caps

Total servings: 6

The **Ingredients** to Use

- ¼ cup of olive oil

- 2 cloves of garlic

- 24 medium mushrooms with the stems removed and kept

- ½ cup of bread crumbs

- ¼ cup of grated Romano

- 6 slices of cooked turkey bacon, crumbled

- ¼ cup of grated Gruyere

- 5 oz of chopped spinach

How to Prepare The Meal

1. Ensure your oven is preheated to 375°F.

2. Grease a cookie sheet and bake your mushrooms on it. Do this with the top of the mushroom cap facing up.

3. Diced the stems of mushroom you kept and your garlic. Place a pan containing olive oil over medium heat, sauté your garlic, crumbled and diced turkey bacon, and mushroom stems for 5 minutes. Throw in your spinach and continue cooking for an additional 3 minutes.

4. In a large bowl place your bread crumbs and Romano in it. Mix them together.

5. Turn the contents of your pan into the bowl and continue mixing. Fill each mushroom cap with this mixture, put them on a baking sheet and bake for another 15 minutes.

41. Mini Lasagna Cups

Total servings: 12

The **Ingredients** to Use

- 24 wrappers of wonton

- 6 oz of ground turkey

- 1 cup of pesto sauce

- 1 cup of low-fat cottage cheese

- 1 ½ cups of shredded Parmesan cheese

- 1 ½ cups of skimmed mozzarella cheese

How to Prepare The Meal

1. Make sure your oven is preheated to 375°F.

2. Spray the openings of a muffin tin with olive oil.

3. In a skillet, cook your turkey until it is brown, and add salt and pepper to your preferred taste.

4. Place a wrapper of wonton into each muffin cup and push down. Place your cheeses, meat, and pesto in layers.

5. Place a wonton wrapper on that layer and continue with more layers.

6. Place what's left of your mozzarella and Parmesan cheese on top of those layers.

7. Bake for 20 minutes. By this time, the cheese should have melted and the wrappers should have turned brown.

8. Remove the lasagna from the tin and let it cool for a bit.

9. Garnish it with basil leaves.

42. Enchiladas Verdes

Total servings: 9

The **Ingredients** to Use

- 1 cup of cotija cheese, grated

- 2 cloves of garlic

- An 8 oz container of Mexican crema

- 3 Serrano peppers

- 1 cup of cilantro leaves

- 2 ¼ pounds of small green tomatillos, husks removed

- ¼ shredded iceberg lettuce

- 1 cup of vegetable oil

- ½ shredded rotisserie chicken with the meat removed

- 9 corn tortillas

- 4 tsp of chicken flavored Knorr bouillon, granulated

- 3 cups of water

How to Prepare The Meal

1. Preheat your griddle to medium-high after covering it with aluminum foil. Toast your garlic for 5 minutes; tomatillos for 15 minutes, and Serrano

peppers for 10 minutes on the griddle. Set them aside in a bowl.

2. Heat a skillet containing oil to 350°F. Fry your tortillas in the oil for about 15 seconds. Turn them with tongs to ensure they are not burnt.

3. Place the peppers, tomatillos, and garlic you had toasted in a blender and mix until it is smooth. Turn this into a saucepan that is placed over medium-high heat, and boil. Dissolve your Knorr bouillon into the contents of the pan and reduce the heat to medium.

4. Cook for 10 minutes. The sauce should have increased in thickness. One at a time, place each of your tortillas in the sauce and leave them to soak for about 10 seconds. Place the shredded chicken, some sauce, and meat into the tortillas and roll them. Place them down with the seam side facing downward. Pour sauce generously over them and add cilantro, Mexican crema, iceberg lettuce, and cotija cheese on top of the tortillas.

5. If you wish, you can repeat this step (sauce and toppings) twice. Your Enchiladas Verdes is ready to serve.

43. Granola Parfaits

Total servings: 4

The **Ingredients** to Use

- 2 cups of low-fat plain yogurt
- 2 ¼ cups of rolled oats (don't use the kind that cooks quickly)
- ⅓ cup of sunflower seeds, shelled and salted
- 1 cup of sweetened coconut, shredded
- ¾ cup of golden raisins
- ¾ cup of almonds, slivered
- ¾ cup of dried cranberries
- ¼ cup of vegetable oil
- 1 cup of honey

How to Prepare The Meal

1. Ensure that your oven is preheated to 375°F.
2. Then, get a large bowl and place the almonds, rolled oats, and coconut in it. Toss them.
3. Get a smaller bowl and add the oil and honey. Whisk them. Turn your coconut mixture into this bowl and mix them.
4. On a baking sheet that has been rimmed, spread this mixture. Make sure they are evenly spread.

Place the baking sheet in a preheated oven and bake for 20 minutes. Once the mixture in the baking sheet has turned a golden brown color, remove from the oven and allow it to cool for another 20 minutes.

5. Place this baked mixture in a large bowl. Next, add your sunflower seeds, cranberries and raisins. This is your granola.

6. In 4 parfait dishes, spoon large amounts of yogurt into each. Also, spoon a large amount of granola to top the yogurt. Pour some honey and repeat the process once more.

44. Pasta Primavera

Total servings: 4

The **Ingredients** to Use

- ¼ cup of basil leaves, shredded
- 1 tbsp of olive oil
- 2 tbsp of parsley leaves, diced
- 3 cloves of garlic, diced
- ½ cup of Parmesan cheese, grated
- 1 red bell pepper that has been cleaned, deseeded, and diced into long strips
- ¾ pound of whole wheat linguine
- ½ pound of asparagus, trimmed and cut
- 6 oz of carrots, peeled and sliced
- 4 oz of button mushrooms, diced
- 1 tbsp of all-purpose flour (dissolve it in 3 tbsp of water)
- ½ cup of milk
- 6 oz of cherry tomatoes
- 1 cup of chicken stock, low-sodium

How to Prepare The Meal

1. Set your stove to medium-high and place a sauté pan containing oil on it. Cook your garlic in it for about 1 minute.

2. Add your peppers to the pan and cook for 3 minutes. Also, add tomatoes, mushrooms, and asparagus and cook for 5 minutes. Add flour and continue stirring. Add milk, chicken stock, pepper, and salt to the pan. Reduce the stove to low and stir some carrots in. Continue cooking for 5 minutes or until the liquid thickens.

3. Cook your linguine according to the instructions on the package. Drain the pasta but keep some of the water. Add sauce and the vegetable to the pasta. Also, add some of the pasta water and cook. Garnish with your grated Parmesan, basil, and parsley.

45. Yogurt and Almond Chicken Curry

Total servings: 6

The **Ingredients** to Use

- 20 grams of coriander, diced

- 2 green chilies, diced

- 100 gram of natural yogurt

- 100 grams of almonds, ground

- 12 chicken thighs, with the skin and bones removed

- 1 medium sized ginger, grated

- 4 tsp of garam masala

- 4 cloves of garlic

- 1 cinnamon stick

- 200 ml of cream

- 2 cardamom pods

- 2 tbsp of vegetable oil

- 3 cloves

- 1 diced onion

- 300 ml of water

How to Prepare The Meal

1. Ensure your oven is preheated to 356°F. Get a bowl and put your chilies, single cream, garlic, ginger, almond, and water.

2. In an oven-proof casserole heat some oil in it. Put cardamom, cinnamon, onion, cloves, and half of your garam masala. Stir and fry for a minute, and then add your paste. Reduce the heat and add some salt. Put the chicken in the casserole and add yogurt.

3. Put it in your preheated oven and bake for 40 minutes. Sprinkle the other half of your garam masala and serve with rice.

Conclusion

The next step is to begin implementing the various methods of relief repented within this book so that you can immediately address the symptoms of acid reflux before they take root. Addressing the symptoms, in this manner, will allow your body to fight off disease like GERD and Barrett's disease as soon as possible rather than at a later time when your body is significantly weaker. Keep in mind that the best method of addressing your symptoms is to consult a medical professional. In this way, you can begin to implement the strategies presented in this book with guidance from a qualified medical professional.

Given that your acid reflux is likely to exist on a ranging spectrum and will most definitely be different for every individual, this book provides methods of addressing your symptoms and ailments in a manner that is applicable and helpful for whichever stage of the reflux you are experiencing. What's more, the 30-day recovery plan is a great way to ensure that your symptoms are staved off for good once you can utilize medical intervention. If, for instance, you are prescribed drugs to mitigate your symptoms, be sure to use the methods outlined in this book in conjunction with the prescribed amount of medication that your doctor has instructed.

Where your health is concerned, being prepared and informed is critical to seeing that you successfully overcome the ailments that are affecting you.

That is precisely why this book is of value. After reading, you are now informed about the intricate aspects of acid reflux and should feel extremely prepared as you move forward in addressing these symptoms.

For this is not truly the end is it, but merely a small step in a forward direction. It is now time to utilize what you have learned going through these pages, and all that the knowledge contained within has to offer. If you or a loved one you know has, has had, or may seem to have a thyroid issue, every tool that is needed to aid them or yourself in the journey forward is now at your fingertips.

Now is when it is time to go see a doctor, to make sure that information is properly communicated. It is never too late, and never a bad idea, especially where the thyroid gland is concerned, to set oneself up with a regular and balanced diet, as well as having a plan for daily exercise in a range of activities.

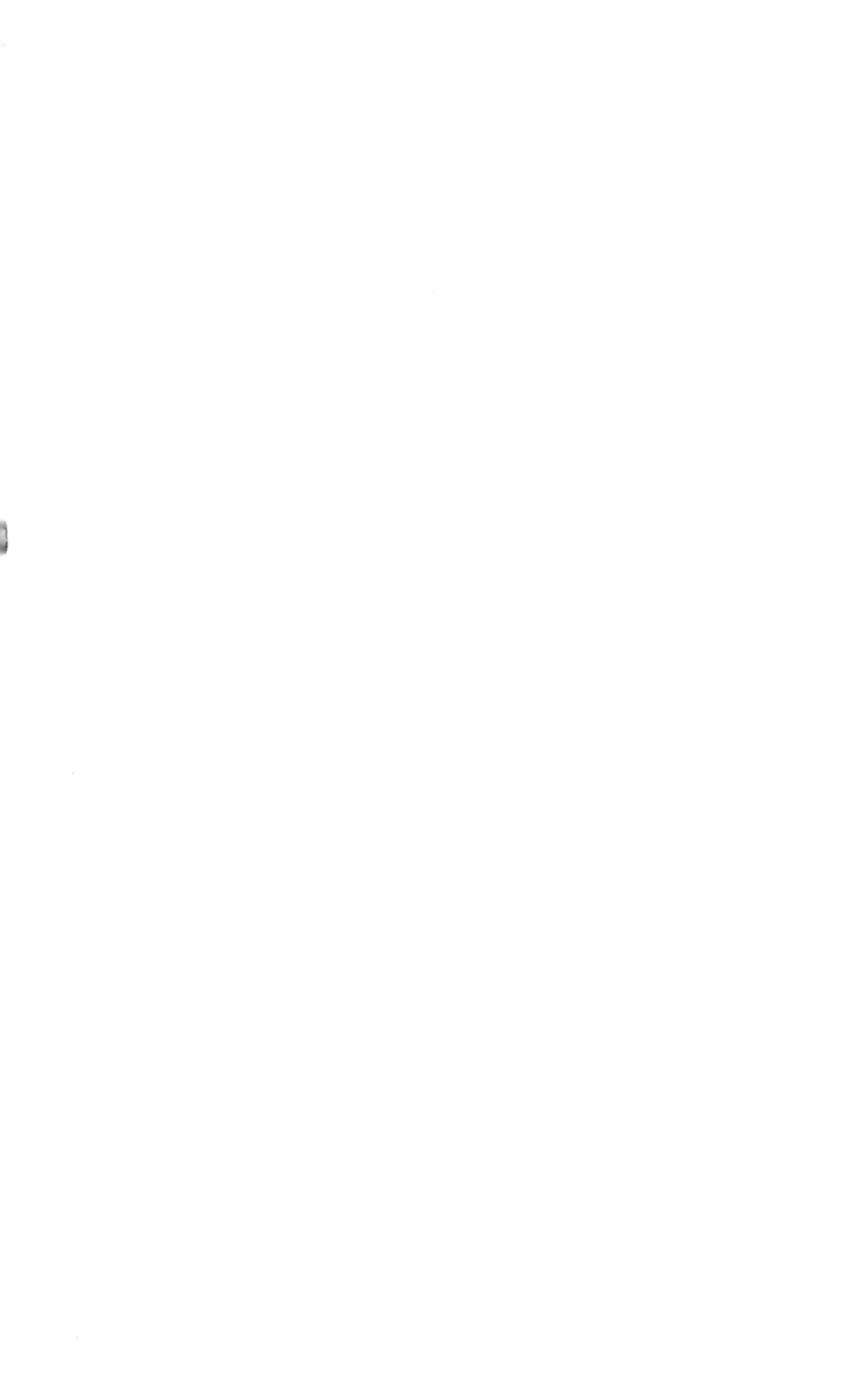

www.ingramcontent.com/pod-product-compliance
Lightning Source LLC
Chambersburg PA
CBHW060323030426
42336CB00011B/1182